Safe Abortion:
Technical and Policy Guidance for Health Systems

TO BE
DISPOSED
BY
AUTHORITY

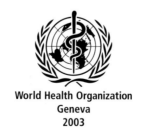

World Health Organization
Geneva
2003

Acknowledgments

The World Health Organization gratefully acknowledges the contribution of those who have collaborated on the elaboration of the publication, and in particular the participants at the WHO Technical Consultation on Safe Abortion held in Geneva in September 2000, for their contributions and subsequent review. The preparation and printing of the publication, and holding of the Technical Consultation, were made possible through financial contributions from the David and Lucille Packard Foundation, the Ford Foundation, the Swedish International Development Cooperation Agency, and the United Kingdom Department for International Development.

World Health Organization
20 Avenue Appia
1211 Geneva 27
Switzerland
Fax: +41-22-791-4171
Email: rhrpublications@who.int
Website: http://www.who.int/reproductive-health/

WHO Library Cataloguing-in-Publication Data

World Health Organization.
  Safe abortion : technical and policy guidance for health systems.

  1.Abortion, Induced - methods 2.Abortion, Induced - standards. 3.Prenatal care - organization and administration 4.Prenatal care - standards 5.Maternal welfare 6.Health policy 7. Guidelines I.Title

  ISBN 92 4 159034 3   (NLM classification: WQ 440)

Designed by Clarus Design, UK

Contents

Safe Abortion: Technical and Policy Guidance for Health Systems

Introduction

In October 2000, at the United Nations Millennium Summit, all countries agreed on the global imperative to reduce poverty and inequities. The need to improve maternal health was identified as one of the key Millennium Development Goals, with a target of reducing levels of maternal mortality by three-quarters between 1990 and 2015.

The causes of maternal deaths are multiple. Women die because complications during labour and delivery go unrecognised or are inadequately managed. They die from diseases such as malaria, that are aggravated by pregnancy. They die because of complications arising early in pregnancy, sometimes even before they are aware of being pregnant, such as ectopic pregnancy. And they die because they seek to end unwanted pregnancies but lack access to appropriate services. Achieving the Millennium Development Goal of improved maternal health and reducing maternal mortality requires actions on all these fronts.

Despite dramatically increased use of contraception over the past three decades, an estimated 40-50 million abortions occur annually, nearly half of them in circumstances that are unsafe. Globally, approximately 13% of all maternal deaths are due to complications of unsafe abortion. In addition to some 70,000 women who die each year, tens of thousands suffer long-term health consequences including infertility. Even where family planning is widely accessible, pregnancies occur due to contraceptive failure, difficulties with use, non use or as a result of incest or rape. Pregnancy may pose a threat to the woman's life or to her physical and mental health. In recognition of such circumstances, nearly all countries in the world have passed laws that permit termination of pregnancy under specified conditions. In some settings, abortion is legal only to save the woman's life; in others, abortion is allowed upon request by the woman. Health systems need to respond accordingly.

The role of the World Health Organization is to develop norms and standards and provide advice to Member States in order to strengthen the capacity of health systems. For over three decades WHO has assisted governments, international agencies and non-governmental organizations to plan and deliver maternal health services, including managing complications of unsafe abortion and providing high-quality family planning services.

At the Special Session of the United Nations General Assembly in June 1999, Governments agreed that "in circumstances where abortion is not against the law, health systems should train and equip health-service providers and should take other measures to ensure that such abortion is safe and accessible. Additional measures should be taken to safeguard women's health."

This document provides guidance to turn this agreement into reality.

Chapter 1

Safe abortion services: the public health challenge

Chapter 1 Summary

- An estimated 46 million pregnancies end in induced abortion each year. Nearly 20 million of these are estimated to be unsafe.

- About 13 per cent of pregnancy-related deaths have been attributed to complications of unsafe abortion, and probably number about 67,000 deaths annually.

- In developing countries, the risk of death following complications of unsafe abortion procedures is several hundred times higher than that of an abortion performed professionally under safe conditions.

- Complications resulting from unsafe abortion contribute to serious sequelae for women's health such as infertility.

- Since no contraceptive is 100 per cent effective, there will continue to be unwanted pregnancies which women may seek to end by induced abortion.

- In almost all countries the law permits abortion to save the woman's life and in most countries abortion is allowed to preserve the physical and mental health of the woman.

- Safe abortion services, as provided by law, therefore need to be available, provided by well-trained health personnel supported by policies, regulations and a health systems infrastructure, including equipment and supplies, so that women can have rapid access to these services.

1 Background

The International Conference on Population and Development (ICPD) in Cairo in 1994 and the Fourth World Conference on Women (FWCW) in Beijing in 1995 both affirmed the human rights of women in the area of reproductive and sexual health. The Cairo Conference agreed that "Reproductive rights embrace certain human rights that are already recognised in national laws, international human rights documents and other consensus documents. These rights rest on the recognition of the basic rights of all couples and individuals to decide freely and responsibly the number, spacing and timing of their children and to have the information and means to do so, and the right to attain the highest standard of sexual and reproductive health." (United Nations 1995, paragraph 7.3).

In Beijing, Governments agreed that "The human rights of women include their right to have control over and decide freely and responsibly on matters related to their sexuality, including sexual and reproductive health, free of coercion, discrimination and violence. Equal relationships between women and men in matters of sexual relations and reproduction, including full respect for the integrity of the person, require mutual respect, consent and shared responsibility for sexual behaviour and its consequences." (United Nations 1996, paragraph 96).

On the subject of abortion in particular, at the Cairo Conference, Governments of the world recognised unsafe abortion as a major public health concern, and pledged their commitment to reducing the need for abortion through expanded and improved family planning services, while at the same time recognising that, in circumstances where not against the law, abortion should be safe (United Nations 1995, paragraph 8.25). One year later, the Beijing Conference affirmed these agreements and also called for Governments to consider reviewing laws containing punitive measures against women who have undergone illegal abortions (United Nations 1996, paragraph 106).

The United Nations General Assembly review and appraisal of the implementation of ICPD in 1999 (ICPD + 5) further agreed that, "in circumstances where abortion is not against the law, health systems should train and equip health-service providers and should take other measures to ensure that such abortion is safe and accessible. Additional measures should be taken to safeguard women's health." (United Nations 1999, paragraph 63.iii).

For many years, the World Health Organization (WHO) and other organisations have elaborated guidelines for the prevention of unsafe abortion and the management of its complications (see Annex 1). This document provides technical guidance to Governments, policy-makers, programme managers and health workers on how to implement paragraph 63.iii cited above.

2   Induced abortion

Of the 210 million pregnancies that occur each year, about 46 million (22 per cent) end in induced abortion and, globally, the vast majority of women are likely to have at least one abortion by the time they are 45 (Alan Guttmacher Institute 1999). Where effective contraceptive methods are available and widely used, the total abortion rate declines sharply (Bongaarts and Westoff 2000), but has nowhere declined to zero for several reasons. First, millions of women and men either do not have access to appropriate contraceptive methods, or do not have adequate information and support to use them effectively. Second, no contraceptive method is 100 per cent effective. Table 1.1 illustrates this point, using estimates calculated for "perfect use" of a method, in which the user always follows instructions for use exactly, and those calculated for "typical use" which takes into account that people do not always manage to use contraceptives perfectly. Third, high rates of violence against women including in the home and in war lead to unwanted pregnancies. Fourth, changing circumstances, such as divorce or other crisis, can result in a wanted pregnancy becoming unwanted.

3   Unsafe abortion

Even if all contraceptive users were to use methods perfectly all the time, there would still be nearly six million accidental pregnancies annually. Thus, even with high rates of contraceptive use, unwanted pregnancies will occur which women may seek to end by induced abortion.

An unsafe abortion is "a procedure for terminating an unwanted pregnancy either by persons lacking the necessary skills or in an environment lacking the minimal medical standards, or both" (World Health Organization 1992). About 20 million, or nearly half, of the induced abortions annually are estimated to be unsafe. Ninety-five per cent of these occur in developing countries (World Health Organization 1998). Globally, there is a ratio of one unsafe abortion for every seven live births (World Health Organization 1998), but in some regions the ratio is much higher. For instance, in Latin America and the Caribbean, there is more than one unsafe abortion for every three live births (World Health Organization 1998).

Table 1.1 Estimated accidental pregnancies resulting from contraceptive failure worldwide (estimates for 1993)

Contraceptive method	Estimated failure rate (perfect use)[1] %	Estimated failure rate (typical use)[1] %	Number of users[2] 000's	Number of accidental pregnancies (perfect use) 000's	Number of accidental pregnancies (typical use) 000's
Female sterilization	0.50	0.50	201,000	1,005	1,005
Male sterilization	0.10	0.15	41,000	41	62
Injectables	0.30	0.30	26,000	78	78
IUD	0.60	0.80	149,000	894	1,192
Pill	0.10	5.00	78,000	78	3,900
Male condom	3.00	14.00	51,000	1,530	7,140
Vaginal barrier	6.00	20.00	4,000	240	800
Periodic abstinence	3.00	25.00	26,000	780	6,500
Withdrawal	4.00	19.00	31,000	1,240	5,890
Total			607,000	5,886	26,567

[1] Trussel (1998) Estimates based on USA data. Failure rates are expressed as percentage of women who will become pregnant during one year while using the method.

[2] United Nations Population Division (2002). Estimated number of women aged 15-49 who are in a marital or consensual union.

3   Unsafe abortion *continued*

About 13 per cent of pregnancy-related deaths have been attributed to complications of unsafe abortion (World Health Organization 1998); when applied to the most recent estimate of maternal deaths worldwide (i.e. 515,000 for the year 1995; World Health Organization 2001), this percentage corresponds to about 67,000 deaths annually. In addition, unsafe abortion is associated with considerable morbidity. For instance, studies indicate that at least one in five women who have an unsafe abortion suffer a reproductive tract infection as a result. Some of these are serious infections, leading to infertility (World Health Organization 1998).

Where access to abortion services is legally restricted, or where the law provides for abortion on many grounds but services are not fully available or are of poor quality, women who have money are nonetheless often able to buy medically competent services from the private sector. But many other women who have unwanted pregnancies are at particular risk of unsafe abortion. They include women who are poor, live in isolated areas, are in vulnerable circumstances (such as refugees or internally displaced women) or are adolescents, especially those who are not married. These women have less access to reproductive health information and services, they are often highly vulnerable to sexual coercion and violence, they may delay seeking abortion, and they are thus more likely to have to rely on unsafe abortion methods and unskilled providers (Bott 2001, Gardner and Blackburn 1996, Mundigo and Indriso 1999).

4   Safe abortion

Almost all the deaths and complications from unsafe abortion are preventable. Procedures and techniques for early induced abortion are simple and safe. When performed by trained health care providers with proper equipment, correct technique and sanitary standards, abortion is one of the safest medical procedures. In countries where women have access to safe services, their likelihood of dying as a result of an abortion performed with modern methods is no more than one per 100,000 procedures (Alan Guttmacher Institute 1999). In developing countries, the risk of death following complications of unsafe abortion procedures is several hundred times higher than that of an abortion performed professionally under safe conditions (World Health Organization 1998). Properly provided services for early abortion save women's lives and avoid the often substantial costs of treating preventable complications of unsafe abortion (Fortney 1981, Tshibangu et al. 1984, Figa-Talamanca et al. 1986, Mpangile et al. 1999).

5   Legal, policy and contextual considerations

In almost all countries, the law permits abortion to save the woman's life (Figure 1.1). In more than three-fifths of countries, abortion is also allowed to preserve the physical and mental health of the woman and, in about 40 per cent, abortion is permitted in cases of rape or incest or fetal impairment. One-third of countries allow abortion on economic or social grounds, and at least one-quarter allow abortion on request (United Nations Population Division 1999). Thus, virtually all countries should have accessible and safe services in place to provide abortion where the law permits.

Nonetheless, in many circumstances where women are legally entitled to have an abortion, safe services are not available for a range of reasons. These include health system problems such as a lack of trained providers or their concentration in urban areas, negative provider attitudes, use of inappropriate or outdated methods of inducing abortion, lack of authorisation for providers or facilities, lack of knowledge of the law or lack of application of the law by providers, complex regulatory requirements, or lack of resources. Broader policy and social factors, such as regulatory or legal requirements; lack of public information about the law and women's rights under the law; lack of awareness about facilities providing abortion or the need to obtain abortion early in pregnancy; family attitudes; stigmatisation and fears about privacy and confidentiality; and the perceived quality of care provided, must also be addressed if safe, legal services are to be accessible.

Health professionals at all levels have ethical and legal obligations to respect women's rights. Working together with the Ministries of Health and Justice, and their professional associations, they can help to clarify the circumstances where abortion is not against the law. They should understand and apply their national law related to abortion, and contribute to the development of regulations, policies and protocols to ensure access to quality services to the extent permitted by law and respecting women's rights to humane and confidential treatment. Ready access to early safe abortion significantly reduces high rates of maternal mortality and morbidity; it prevents the costs currently imposed by unsafe abortion on health systems; it provides care for women who clearly are not yet well enough served by family planning programmes or for whom contraception has failed.

Figure 1.1 Grounds on which abortion is permitted – percentage of countries

Ground	Percentage
To save a woman's life	98%
To preserve physical health	63%
To preserve mental health	62%
Rape or incest	43%
Fetal impairment	39%
Economic or social reasons	33%
On request	27%

Source: United Nations Population Division 1999

6 The challenge – making safe services available

Making abortion safe and accessible to the full extent of the law requires training health personnel so that they are conversant with national laws and regulations as well as with technical procedures, ensuring equipment and supplies, and designing protocols, regulations and policies that promote access to quality abortion services. The chapters which follow make recommendations on each of these, based on available evidence and experience, and guided by the principles agreed upon in ICPD, FWCW, ICPD+5 and FWCW+5, and in conformity with international human rights. Given that abortion is legal for certain indications in most countries of the world, there is considerable scope in almost every country – both developed and developing – to apply the guidance put forth in this document.

- Chapter 2, "Clinical care for women undergoing abortion", reviews clinical aspects of providing high-quality abortion services, including diagnosis of pregnancy, provision of information and counselling, selection and provision of an appropriate abortion method, and care after abortion. It describes recommended abortion methods and the characteristics that influence their safety, efficacy and optimal use.

- Chapter 3, "Putting services in place", provides guidance on the essential elements needed to put good-quality, legal abortion services in place. Topics discussed include needs assessment, national norms and standards, elements of care at each level of the health system, ensuring provider skills and performance, certification and licensing, monitoring and evaluation, and financing.

- Chapter 4, "Legal and policy considerations", lays out a policy framework to ensure access to safe abortion services to the full extent of the law. Topics include legal grounds for abortion, creating an enabling policy context and removing unnecessary barriers to care.

Further resources and readings are included in Annex 1, to which readers can refer for more in-depth information on topics discussed in the monograph. Annex 2 provides the relevant text from international consensus documents, and Annexes 3 and 4 provide further details about equipment needed and about contraception after abortion, respectively.

References

Alan Guttmacher Institute. (1999) *Sharing responsibility: women, society & abortion worldwide.* New York and Washington DC, The Alan Guttmacher Institute.

Bongaarts J and Westoff CF. (2000) The potential role of contraception in reducing abortion. *Studies in Family Planning* 31:193-202.

Bott S. (2001) Unwanted pregnancy and induced abortion among adolescents in developing countries: findings from WHO case studies. In: Puri CP and Van Look PFA (eds). *Sexual and reproductive health: recent advances, future directions.* New Delhi, New Age International (P) Limited, Volume 1, 351-366.

Figa-Talamanca I, Sinnathuray TA, Yusof K, Fong CK, Palan VT, Adeeb N, Nylander P, Onifade A, Akin A and Bertan M. (1986) Illegal abortion: an attempt to assess its costs to the health services and its incidence in the community. *International Journal of Health Services* 16:375-389.

Fortney JA. (1981) The use of hospital resources to treat incomplete abortions: examples from Latin America. *Public Health Reports* 96:574-579.

Gardner R and Blackburn R. (1996) People who move: new reproductive health focus. *Population Reports* Series J, No. 45.

Mpangile GS, Leshabari MT and Kihwele DJ. (1999) Induced abortion in Dar es Salaam, Tanzania: the plight of adolescents. In: Mundigo AI and Indriso C. (eds). *Abortion in the developing world.* New Delhi, Vistaar Publications for the World Health Organization, pp. 387-403.

Mundigo AI and Indriso C. (eds). (1999) *Abortion in the developing world.* New Delhi, Vistaar Publications for the World Health Organization.

Trussell J. (1998) Contraceptive efficacy. In: Hatcher RA, Trussell J, Stewart F, Cates W Jr, Stewart GK, Guest F and Kowal D (eds). *Contraceptive technology (17th revised edition).* New York, Ardent Media Inc., pp. 779-844.

Tshibangu K, Ntabona B, Liselele-Bolemba L and Mbiye K. (1984) Avortement clandestin, problème de santé publique à Kinshasa. [Illicit abortion, a public health problem in Kinshasa (Zaire)] *Journal de Gynécologie, Obstétrique et Biologie de la Reproduction (Paris)* 13:759-763.

United Nations. (1995) *Report of the International Conference on Population and Development, Cairo, 5-13 September 1994.* New York, United Nations. (Sales No. 95.XIII.18)

United Nations. (1996) *Report of the Fourth World Conference on Women, Beijing, 4-15 September 1995.* New York, United Nations. (Sales No. 96.IV.13)

United Nations. (1999) *Key actions for the further implementation of the Programme of Action of the International Conference on Population and Development.* New York, United Nations. (A/S-21/5/Add.1)

United Nations Population Division. (1999) *World abortion policies 1999.* New York, United Nations. Population Division (ST/ESA/SER.A/178).

United Nations Population Division. (2002) *World contraceptive use 2001.* New York, United Nations (Sales No. E.02.XIII.7).

World Health Organization. (1992) *The prevention and management of unsafe abortion. Report of a Technical Working Group.* Geneva, World Health Organization. (WHO/MSM/92.5)

World Health Organization. (1998) *Unsafe abortion: global and regional estimates of incidence of and mortality due to unsafe abortion with a listing of available country data.* Geneva, World Health Organization. (WHO/RHT/MSM/97.16)

World Health Organization. (2001) *Maternal mortality in 1995: estimates developed by WHO, UNICEF, UNFPA.* Geneva, World Health Organization. (WHO/RHR/01.9)

Chapter **2** Clinical care for women undergoing abortion

Chapter 2 Summary

Pre-abortion care

- Determining the length of pregnancy is a critical factor in selecting the most appropriate abortion method. Bimanual pelvic examination and recognition of other symptoms of pregnancy is usually adequate. Laboratory or ultrasound testing may be used for confirmation.

- In areas where anaemia is prevalent, measuring haemoglobin or haematocrit levels will enable prompt response in case of complications potentially requiring blood transfusion.

- Routine use of antibiotics at the time of abortion reduces the post-procedural risk of infection. However, abortion should not be denied where prophylactic antibiotics are not available.

- Complete, accurate and easy-to-understand information about the procedure and what to expect during and afterwards must be given to the woman, as well as voluntary counselling about options available to her to help her make informed decisions.

Methods of abortion

- The following methods are preferred for early (first trimester) abortion:

  - Manual or electric vacuum aspiration, for up to 12 completed weeks since the woman's last menstrual period;

  - Medical method of abortion – a combination of mifepristone followed by a prostaglandin such as misoprostol or gemeprost, for up to 9 completed weeks since last menstrual period. Misoprostol is the prostaglandin of choice for most settings since it is cheap and does not require refrigeration.

- Dilatation and curettage (D&C) should be used only where vacuum aspiration or medical methods of abortion are not available.

- For pregnancies of more than 12 completed weeks since the woman's last menstrual period, the following methods are preferred:

  - Dilatation and evacuation (D&E), using vacuum aspiration and forceps;

  - Mifepristone followed by repeated doses of a prostaglandin such as misoprostol or gemeprost;

  - Prostaglandins alone (misoprostol or gemeprost), in repeated doses.

- Cervical preparation before surgical abortion is recommended for durations of pregnancy over 9 completed weeks for nulliparous women, for women younger than 18 years old, and for all women with durations of pregnancy over 12 completed weeks.

- Medication for pain management should always be offered. In most cases, analgesics, local anaesthesia and/or mild sedation supplemented by verbal support are sufficient.

- Local anaesthesia, such as lidocaine injected around the cervix, should be used to alleviate women's discomfort where mechanical cervical dilatation is required for surgical abortion. General anaesthesia is not recommended for abortion as it has been associated with higher rates of complications than local anaesthesia.

- Universal precautions for infection control should be used, as with the care of all patients at all times, to reduce the risk of transmission of bloodborne infections including HIV.

Follow-up

- For surgical abortion, women can leave the health care facility as soon as they feel able and their vital signs are normal.

- For surgical methods, women should ideally have a follow-up visit 7-10 days after the procedure.

- For medical methods of abortion, if abortion is not complete before they leave the health facility, women should return after 10-15 days for confirmation that the abortion has been completed.

- Before they leave the health care facility, all women should receive information on contraception and, for those who want them, contraceptives or referral to contraceptive services.

- Women should receive oral and written instructions about how to care for themselves after leaving the health care facility, about how much bleeding to expect, and about recognizing complications and how to seek help for them.

Definitions used in this document

Surgical methods of abortion
- Use of transcervical procedures for terminating pregnancy, including vacuum aspiration, dilatation & curettage (D&C), and dilatation and evacuation (D&E).

Medical methods of abortion
- Use of pharmacological drugs to terminate pregnancy. Sometimes the term "non-surgical abortion" is also used.

Duration of pregnancy
- The number of completed days or weeks since the first day of the woman's last normal menstrual period.

Menstrual regulation
- Early uterine evacuation without laboratory or ultrasound confirmation of pregnancy for women who report delayed menses.

1   Pre-abortion care

The first steps in providing abortion care are to establish that the woman is indeed pregnant and, if so, to estimate the duration of the pregnancy and confirm that the pregnancy is intrauterine. The risks associated with induced abortion, though small when abortion is properly performed, increase with the duration of pregnancy (Grimes and Cates 1979). Thus, determination of the length of pregnancy is a critical factor in selecting the most appropriate abortion method.

Every health service delivery point should have staff trained and competent to take the woman's history and perform a bimanual pelvic examination. Health centres not staffed and equipped to provide induced abortion must be able to refer women promptly to the nearest services. Staff should also be competent to offer counselling to help the woman consider her options (see section 1.10.1).

1.1   PATIENT HISTORY

Most women begin to suspect that they are pregnant when a menstrual period is late. The woman should be asked about the first day of her last menstrual period (LMP), i.e. the first day of bleeding and whether the menses was normal. Women may experience amenorrhoea for reasons other than pregnancy, however, and some women who are pregnant may not report having missed a period. For example, women who are breastfeeding may become pregnant before their first postpartum menses. Some women may experience non-menstrual bleeding in early pregnancy, and this can be a cause of missing or misdating pregnancy. Other symptoms that women commonly report in early pregnancy include breast tenderness and engorgement, nausea sometimes accompanied by vomiting, fatigue, changes in appetite and increased frequency of urination.

1.2   PHYSICAL EXAMINATION

Health providers must confirm pregnancy and estimate its duration by a bimanual pelvic examination. While many health workers have been trained to assess the length of pregnancy in order to provide prenatal care, many are not experienced in diagnosing very early pregnancy or accurately estimating length of pregnancy during the first trimester. Hence, additional training is often required for staff who are to provide abortion services (see Chapter 3).

Signs of pregnancy detectable during a bimanual pelvic examination as early as 6 to 8 weeks of pregnancy include softening of the cervical isthmus and softening and enlargement of the uterus. A uterus in a pregnant woman that is smaller than expected could be due to a pregnancy that is less advanced than estimated from the date of LMP, an ectopic pregnancy, or a missed abortion; and a larger than expected uterus may indicate a pregnancy that is more advanced than calculated from the date of LMP, a multiple pregnancy, the presence of uterine fibroids, or a molar pregnancy.

1   Pre-abortion care *continued*

During the physical examination, the health worker should also assess whether the uterus is anteverted, retroverted or otherwise positioned in a way that might affect assessment of the length of pregnancy or complicate a surgical abortion. Providers should be trained to recognize signs of sexually transmitted infections (STIs) and other reproductive tract infections (RTIs) as well as other conditions such as anaemia or malaria that may require additional service procedures or referral for medical attention. In cases where serious cervical pathology is observed, the woman should be referred to appropriate facilities for further examination.

1.3   LABORATORY TESTING

In most cases, providers only require the information obtained from the woman's history and from a physical examination to confirm the pregnancy and estimate its length. Laboratory testing for pregnancy may not be needed, unless the typical signs of pregnancy are not clearly present and the provider is unsure whether the woman is pregnant. However, obtaining such tests should not hinder or delay uterine evacuation.

Measuring haemoglobin or haematocrit levels to detect anaemia in areas where it is prevalent, enables the provider to initiate treatment and be prepared if haemorrhage occurs at the time of or following the abortion procedure.

Tests for ABO and Rhesus (Rh) blood group typing should be provided where feasible, especially at higher-level referral centres, in case of complications that might require blood transfusion (see 2.5.2.3 below).

1.4   ULTRASOUND SCANNING

Ultrasound scanning is not necessary for the provision of early abortion (RCOG 2000). Where it is available, ultrasound can aid the detection of ectopic pregnancies beyond about 6 weeks of pregnancy. Some providers find the technology helpful before or during abortion procedures at later stages of pregnancy. Where ultrasound is used, service delivery sites should, if possible, provide separate areas where women seeking abortion can be scanned, away from those receiving prenatal care.

1.5   PRE-EXISTING CONDITIONS

In addition to confirming and estimating the duration of pregnancy, health workers should obtain a full medical history and assess other factors that may affect the provision of abortion. These include: bleeding disorders, allergies to any medication to be used during the abortion, and information about any drugs the woman is taking that could interact with those to be used during the procedure.

From a clinical point of view, presence of HIV infection in a woman undergoing abortion requires the same precautions as for other medical/surgical interventions (see 2.5.1 below). If the woman is known to be HIV-positive, she may need special counselling (see 1.10.1).

1.6 REPRODUCTIVE TRACT INFECTIONS (RTIs)

The presence of infection in the lower reproductive tract at the time of abortion is a risk factor for post-procedural RTIs (Penney et al. 1998). The routine use of antibiotics at the time of abortion has been reported to reduce the post-procedural risk of infection by half (Sawaya et al. 1996). However, where antibiotics are not available for prophylactic use, abortion can be performed. In any case, strict observation of cleaning and disinfection procedures plays an essential role in preventing post-procedural infection (see section 2.5.1).

If clinical signs indicate infection, the woman should be treated immediately with antibiotics and abortion can then be carried out. Where laboratory testing for RTIs is routinely performed, and if there are no visible signs of infection, abortion should not be delayed to wait for the test results.

1.7 ECTOPIC PREGNANCY

Ectopic pregnancy can be life-threatening. Signs that might indicate extrauterine pregnancy include uterine size smaller than expected for the estimated length of pregnancy and lower abdominal pain, especially if accompanied by vaginal bleeding and spotting, dizziness or fainting, pallor and, in some women, an adnexal mass. If ectopic pregnancy is suspected, it is essential to confirm diagnosis immediately and initiate treatment or transfer the woman as soon as possible to a facility that has the capacity to confirm diagnosis and initiate treatment (see World Health Organization 2000a for treatment details).

It should be noted that it is more difficult to diagnose an ectopic pregnancy during and after medical methods of abortion due to similarity of symptoms. Therefore, if medical methods of abortion are being used without prior confirmation that the pregnancy is intrauterine, and the woman has severe and intensifying pain after the procedure, she should undergo assessment for ectopic pregnancy.

1.8 RH-ISOIMMUNISATION

Passive immunisation of all Rh-negative women with Rh-immunoglobulin within 72 hours after abortion was recommended in the USA in 1961 (Finn et al. 1961), yet there is still no conclusive evidence about the need for this measure after first-trimester induced abortion. Where Rh-immunoglobulin is routinely provided in the facility to Rh-negative women, it should be administered at the time of the abortion procedure. For women using medical methods of abortion, administration of Rh-immunoglobulin has been recommended at the time of the prostaglandin administration (Urquhart and Templeton 1990).

1.9   CERVICAL CYTOLOGY

Some sites may also offer women cervical smears and other reproductive health services. An abortion request may be an opportunity for assessing cervical cytology of women, especially in settings where there is a high prevalence of cervical cancer and STIs. However, accepting such services must never be a condition for a woman to obtain an abortion and these services are not required in order to perform abortion safely.

1.10   INFORMATION AND COUNSELLING

The provision of information is an essential part of good-quality abortion services. Information must be complete, accurate and easy to understand, and be given in a way that respects the woman's privacy and confidentiality. Chapter 3 gives details about training and other provider requirements related to provision of information and counselling, including ethical standards.

1.10.1   Decision-making counselling

Counselling can be very important in helping the woman consider her options and ensure that she can make a decision free from pressure. Counselling should be voluntary, confidential and provided by a trained person.

If the woman opts for abortion, the health worker should explain any legal requirements for obtaining it. The woman should be given as much time as she needs to make a decision, even if it means returning to the clinic later. However, the greater safety and effectiveness of early abortion should be explained. The health worker should also provide information for women who decide to carry the pregnancy to term and/or consider adoption, including referral as appropriate.

In some circumstances the woman may be under pressure from her partner or other family members to have an abortion. Unmarried adolescents and women who are HIV-infected may be particularly vulnerable to such pressure. All women who are known to be HIV-infected need to know the risks of pregnancy to their own health and the risks of transmission of the virus to their infants. They also need to know about treatments available for themselves and for preventing transmission to infants in order to make an informed decision about whether to continue with the pregnancy or have it terminated, where permitted by law. They may also request additional counselling (World Health Organization 1999). If health workers suspect coercion, they should talk with the woman alone, or refer her for additional counselling. If staff know or suspect that the woman has been subjected to sexual violence or abuse, they should refer her for other counselling and treatment services as appropriate. Managers should ensure that all staff know about the availability of such resources in the health system and the community (see Chapter 3).

1.10.2　Information on abortion procedures

At a minimum, a woman must be given information on:

- what will be done during and after the procedure;

- what she is likely to experience
  (e.g. menstrual-like cramps, pain and bleeding);

- how long the procedure will take;

- what pain management can be made
  available to her;

- risks and complications associated with the method;

- when she will be able to resume her normal
  activities, including sexual intercourse; and

- follow-up care.

If a choice of abortion methods is available, providers should be trained to give women clear information about which methods are appropriate, based on the length of pregnancy and the woman's medical condition and potential risk factors.

1.10.3　Contraceptive information and services

Provision of contraceptive information and services is an essential part of abortion care as it helps the woman avoid unintended pregnancies in the future.

Every woman should be informed that ovulation can return as early as about two weeks after abortion (Cameron and Baird 1988), putting her at risk of pregnancy unless an effective contraceptive method is used. She should be given accurate information to assist her in choosing the most appropriate contraceptive method to meet her needs. If the woman is seeking an abortion following what she considers to be a contraceptive failure, the provider should discuss whether the method may have been used incorrectly and how to correct its use, or whether it may be appropriate for her to change to a different method (for discussion on specific methods, see section 3.2 and Annex 4). The final selection of a method, however, must be the woman's alone.

A woman's acceptance of a contraceptive method must never be a precondition for providing her an abortion.

Figure 2.1 **Methods of abortion**

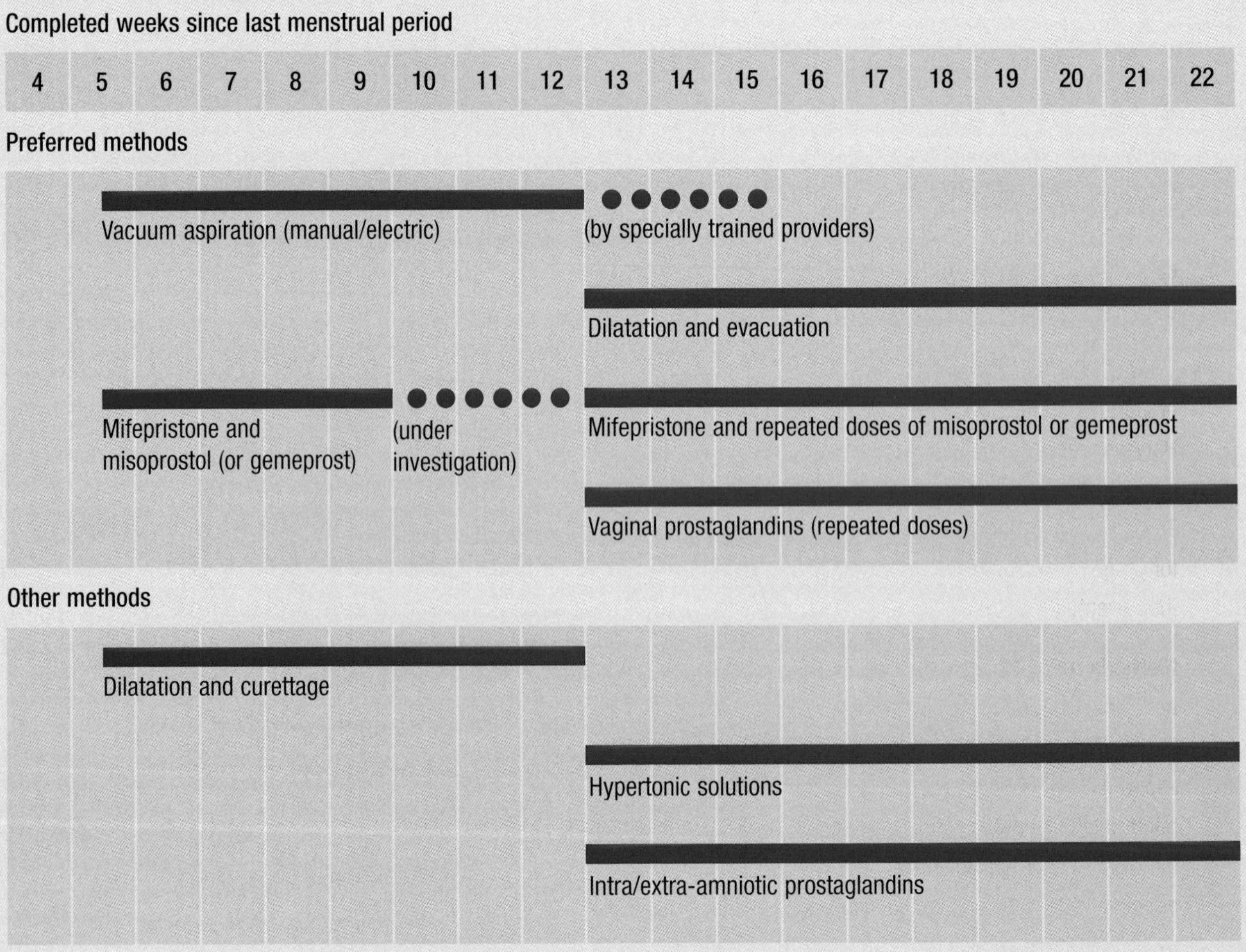

Completed weeks since last menstrual period

4	5	6	7	8	9	10	11	12	13	14	15	16	17	18	19	20	21	22

Preferred methods

Vacuum aspiration (manual/electric)   (by specially trained providers)

Dilatation and evacuation

Mifepristone and misoprostol (or gemeprost)   (under investigation)   Mifepristone and repeated doses of misoprostol or gemeprost

Vaginal prostaglandins (repeated doses)

Other methods

Dilatation and curettage

Hypertonic solutions

Intra/extra-amniotic prostaglandins

2   Methods of abortion

SUMMARY

Figure 2.1 summarises the methods of abortion that are the most appropriate at different stages of pregnancy, based on established protocols used worldwide. It is indicative rather than prescriptive with regard to the time limits. For example, most trained providers can safely undertake vacuum aspiration up to 12 completed weeks of pregnancy, while others with special training, sufficient experience and access to appropriately-sized cannulae can use this procedure safely up to 15 completed weeks (RCOG 2000).

The availability of safe and effective medical methods of inducing abortion remains limited at present. However, rapid development and ongoing research may lead to their wider introduction in the near future. The use of these drugs is therefore discussed in order for programme planners and managers to prepare for their eventual introduction in a systematic manner.

Methods up to 12 completed weeks since last menstrual period

The preferred methods are manual or electric vacuum aspiration, or medical methods using a combination of mifepristone followed by a prostaglandin. Mifepristone followed by a prostaglandin has been shown safe and effective up to 9 completed weeks of pregnancy, and the safety and effectiveness of the regimen between 9 and 12 completed weeks is under investigation.

The use of medical methods of abortion requires the back-up of vacuum aspiration on site or through referral in case of failed or incomplete abortion. Dilatation and curettage (D&C) should be used only where none of the above methods are available. Health managers and policy-makers should make all possible efforts to replace sharp curettage (D&C) with vacuum aspiration.

Methods after 12 completed weeks since last menstrual period

A number of situations give rise to the need for abortion services later in pregnancy, and all levels of the health system should be able to refer women to centres that have the capacity to perform later abortions safely. The diagnosis of fetal abnormalities usually does not occur until after 12 weeks of pregnancy, and serious cardiovascular disease or cancer requiring aggressive treatment for the woman, for example, can necessitate later abortion for medical reasons. Some women, particularly adolescents, cannot easily obtain early care or they delay accessing services. This may be due to the woman's lack of knowledge about conditions under which abortion is permitted, lack of information about or access to health care services, financial constraints, inability to recognize the signs of pregnancy, irregular menses, initial ambivalence about having an abortion, health concerns that arise after the first trimester, family conflict or a change in life circumstances that makes a previously wanted pregnancy no longer feasible.

The preferred medical method for abortions after 12 completed weeks since last menstrual period is mifepristone followed by repeated doses of a prostaglandin such as misoprostol or gemeprost. The preferred surgical method is dilatation and evacuation (D&E), using vacuum aspiration and forceps.

2.1   CERVICAL PREPARATION

Cervical preparation (or priming) using osmotic dilators or pharmacologic agents is commonly used in some countries before first-trimester surgical abortions because it makes the abortion procedure quicker and easier to perform and reduces the incidence of common immediate complications in abortions performed after 9 completed weeks of gestation (World Health Organization 1997). Cervical priming before surgical abortion is especially beneficial for certain women, such as those with cervical anomalies or previous surgery, young women and those with advanced pregnancies, who have a higher risk of cervical injury or uterine perforation that may cause haemorrhage (Grimes et al. 1984, Schulz et al. 1983). However, cervical preparation has some disadvantages, including the extra cost and time required. It is therefore recommended for durations of pregnancy over 9 completed weeks for nulliparous women, for women younger than 18 years old and for all women with durations of pregnancy over 12 completed weeks (RCOG 2000, World Health Organization 1997).

Recent research suggests vaginal administration of 400µg misoprostol 3 to 4 hours before the operation has been found to be effective (Singh et al. 1998). Oral administration of 400µg misoprostol 3 to 4 hours before the procedure is also appropriate for cervical priming (Ngai et al. 1999). Other effective regimens are 200mg mifepristone taken orally 36 hours before the procedure (World Health Organization Task Force on Post-ovulatory Methods of Fertility Regulation 1994) or 1mg gemeprost vaginally administered 3 hours before the procedure (Henshaw and Templeton 1991).

2.2   PAIN MANAGEMENT

Most women report some degree of pain with abortion. The factors associated with pain during surgical abortion with local anaesthesia have been evaluated in several observational studies. The degree of the pain varies with the age of the woman, length of pregnancy, amount of cervical dilatation and the fearfulness of the woman (Smith et al. 1979). Prior vaginal delivery has been found to be a decreasing factor (Borgatta and Nickinovich 1997). Time interval less than 2 minutes between administration of the local anaesthetic and the beginning of the procedure, lack of choice between local and general anaesthesia, and a history of frequent use of analgesics have also been reported to contribute to increased pain (Donati et al. 1996).

Providing adequate pain management does not require a large investment in drugs, equipment or training. Neglecting this important element needlessly increases women's anxiety and discomfort and seriously compromises quality of care.

Counselling and sympathetic treatment is likely to reduce women's fears and perceptions of pain (Solo 2000). The person performing the procedure and other staff present should be friendly and reassuring. Where feasible, and if the woman wishes, it may also be helpful for the woman's husband or partner, a family member or friend to remain with her during the procedure. However, these approaches should not be seen as a replacement for medical pain alleviation.

2.2.1 Medication for pain

Medication for pain management should always be offered. Three types of drugs, either singly or in combination, are used to manage pain during abortion: analgesics, which alleviate the sensation of pain; tranquillizers, which reduce anxiety; and anaesthetics, which numb physical sensation. In most cases, analgesics, local anaesthesia and/or mild sedation supplemented by verbal support, are sufficient. Most of these drugs are comparatively inexpensive.

Non-narcotic analgesics included on WHO's Model List of Essential Medicines such as non-steroidal anti-inflammatory agents are usually sufficient to reduce pain associated with both surgical and medical methods of abortion, including cramping (Suprapto and Reed 1984, Matambo et al. 1999). Paracetamol was found to be ineffective to relieve post-procedural pain in three randomized control trials (Cade and Ashley 1993, Hein et al. 1999, Dahl et al. 2000).

For surgical abortion, preoperative administration of tranquillizers, such as diazepam can reduce fear and induce relaxation, making the procedure easier for both the woman and the provider. Such drugs can cause amnesia, which some women may want, but they may also induce drowsiness and delay ambulation. Supplemental use of narcotic analgesics may also be appropriate, though the possibility of complications such as respiratory depression means that resuscitation capability and narcotic reversal agents must be available.

2.2.2 Anaesthesia

Where mechanical cervical dilatation is required for surgical abortion, a paracervical block, using a local anaesthetic such as the rapidly acting lidocaine, injected beneath the cervical mucosa at the "four quadrant" positions around the cervix should be used to alleviate women's discomfort. Advantages of using local rather than general anaesthesia include a faster recovery time and the fact that the woman remains conscious and hence is able to alert the provider to problems that might arise. Injection of local anaesthetic must be done skillfully, to avoid intravenous introduction of the drug. The use of local anaesthesia with vacuum aspiration has been proved to be safe and effective (Thonneau et al. 1998).

General anaesthesia is not recommended for abortion and increases the clinical risks (Lawson et al. 1994, MacKay et al. 1985, Osborn et al. 1990). It has been associated with higher rates of haemorrhage than local anaesthesia (Grimes and Cates 1979). Use of general anaesthesia increases costs for both the health care facility and the woman, particularly as some hospital policies unnecessarily require women receiving it to stay overnight. Nevertheless, some women prefer general anaesthesia, and its use may also be preferable from the provider's perspective during difficult procedures. Any facility that offers general anaesthesia must have the specialized equipment and staff skilled to administer it and to handle any complications.

2.3   SURGICAL ABORTION

2.3.1   Vacuum aspiration

The preferred surgical technique for abortion up to 12 completed weeks of pregnancy is vacuum aspiration. Some providers, depending on their training and experience and the particular case, are able to use vacuum aspiration up to 15 completed weeks. The high efficacy of vacuum aspiration has been well established in several randomized control trials. Complete abortion rates between 95% and 100% are reported (Greenslade et al. 1993). Electric and manual vacuum technologies appear to be equally effective (Westfall et al. 1998).

Vacuum aspiration involves the evacuation of the contents of the uterus through a plastic or metal cannula, attached to a vacuum source. Electric vacuum aspiration (EVA) employs an electric vacuum pump. With manual vacuum aspiration (MVA), the vacuum is created using a hand-held, hand-activated, plastic 60ml aspirator (also called a syringe). Available aspirators accommodate different sizes of plastic cannulae, ranging from 4 to at least 12mm in diameter. Some cannulae and most aspirators are re-usable after being cleaned and high-level disinfected or sterilized. Foot-operated mechanical pumps are also available.

Depending on the duration of pregnancy, abortion with vacuum aspiration takes from 3 to 10 minutes to complete and can be performed on an outpatient basis, using analgesics and/or local anaesthesia. In very early pregnancy, the cannula may be inserted without prior dilatation of the cervix. Usually, however, dilatation using mechanical or osmotic dilators, alone or in combination with a prostaglandin, or cervical priming with pharmacological agents such as mifepristone or a prostaglandin (misoprostol or gemeprost), is required before insertion of the cannula.

Most women who have first-trimester abortions with local anaesthesia feel well enough to leave the health care facility after observation for about 30 minutes in a recovery room. Longer recovery periods are generally needed for abortions performed later in pregnancy and when sedation or general anaesthesia has been used.

Vacuum aspiration is a very safe procedure. A study of 170,000 first trimester abortions carried out in New York City, USA (the majority by vacuum aspiration) reported that less than 0.1% of the women experienced serious complications requiring hospitalization (Hakim-Elahi et al. 1990). Though rare, complications with vacuum aspiration can include pelvic infection, excessive bleeding, cervical injury, incomplete evacuation, uterine perforation, anaesthesia complications and ongoing pregnancy (Grimes and Cates 1979). Abdominal cramping or pain and menstrual-like bleeding are side-effects of any abortion procedure.

2.3.2   Dilatation and curettage

Dilatation and curettage (D&C), also known as "sharp curettage", involves dilating the cervix with mechanical dilators or pharmacological agents and using sharp metal curettes to scrape the walls of the uterus.

Dilatation and curettage is less safe than vacuum aspiration (Cates et al. 2000) and considerably more painful for women (Grimes et al. 1977). Vacuum aspiration has replaced D&C in routine use in most industrialized countries and in many others. The rates of major complications of D&C are two to three times higher than those of vacuum aspiration (Grimes and Cates 1979). A randomized controlled trial comparing D&C with vacuum aspiration found that, up to 10 weeks since LMP, vacuum aspiration is quicker and associated with less blood loss than D&C (Lean et al. 1976).

Table 2.1 summarizes the requirements for vacuum aspiration and D&C. Where D&C is currently practiced, all possible efforts should be made to replace it with vacuum aspiration, to improve the safety and quality of care. Where no abortion-related services are currently offered, vacuum aspiration should be introduced rather than D&C. At sites where D&C continues to be used, managers must ensure that proper pain management procedures are followed, and that staff are well-trained and receive adequate supervised clinical practice to maintain their skills.

2.3.3   Dilatation and evacuation

Dilatation and evacuation (D&E) is used from about 12 completed weeks of pregnancy. It is the safest and most effective surgical technique for later abortion where skilled, experienced providers are available (RCOG 2000). D&E requires preparing the cervix with mifepristone, a prostaglandin such as misoprostol, or laminaria or similar hydrophilic dilator; dilating the cervix; and evacuating the uterus using electric vacuum aspiration with 14-16mm diameter cannulae and forceps. Depending on the duration of pregnancy, adequate dilatation can require anything from two hours to a full day. Many providers find the use of ultrasound helpful during D&E procedures, but it is not essential.

Table 2.1 **Requirements for vacuum aspiration and dilatation & curettage**

Characteristic	Vacuum Aspiration	Dilatation & Curettage
Location	Examination room, general operating room or ob/gyn operating room	General operating room or ob/gyn operating room
Pain management	Mild sedation, analgesia, and/or local anaesthesia	Heavy or mild sedation, analgesia, and/or local anaesthesia
Level of provider	Gynaecologist, trained general physician, trained mid-level provider	Gynaecologist, trained general physician

Adapted from Greenslade et al. 1993

2 Methods of abortion *continued*

A randomized controlled trial comparing D&E with intra-amniotic instillation of the older prostaglandin $PGF_{2\alpha}$ found D&E to be faster, safer and more acceptable at least through about 18 weeks of pregnancy (Grimes et al. 1980). D&E has not been compared to the newer medical methods such as mifepristone with repeated doses of misoprostol. If providers do not have adequate supervised training and a case-load sufficient to maintain their skills in D&E, then medical methods should be used.

A D&E procedure can usually be performed with only a paracervical block and mild analgesia, and the procedure can thus be performed on an outpatient basis. However, sites offering this procedure should be equipped and have personnel trained to administer conscious sedation or deep sedation, if required. General anaesthesia is not required and can increase risk (see 2.2.2 above). A D&E procedure usually takes no more than 30 minutes to perform. Clinic staff and women undergoing the procedure should expect more post-operative discharge, including bleeding, than after a first-trimester abortion. Staff should also be trained to provide specialized counselling for second-trimester abortion patients.

2.3.4 Other surgical methods of abortion for use in later pregnancy

Major operations should not be used as primary methods of abortion. Hysterotomy has no role in contemporary abortion practice since its morbidity, mortality and cost are markedly higher than with D&E or medical methods of abortion. Similarly, hysterectomy should not be used except for women with conditions that would warrant the operation independently.

2.3.5 Tissue examination following surgical abortion

After surgical methods of abortion, immediate examination of the products of conception is important to exclude the possibility of ectopic pregnancy.

With MVA, after about 6 completed weeks of pregnancy, trained providers can usually visually identify the products of conception, specifically chorionic villi. If the aspirate does not contain the expected products of conception, ectopic pregnancy should be suspected and the woman should undergo further evaluation, as discussed earlier (see 1.7). In addition, providers need to be alert to appearances suggestive of molar pregnancy. If the contents of the aspirate do not conform to the estimated length of pregnancy, health workers should consider the possibility of incomplete abortion. Routine analysis of the products of conception by a pathology laboratory is not essential.

2.4 MEDICAL METHODS OF ABORTION

Medical methods of abortion have been proved to be safe and effective (Ashok et al. 1998a, Peyron et al. 1993, Schaff et al. 1999, Spitz et al. 1998, Trussell and Ellertson 1999, Urquhart et al. 1997, Winikoff et al. 1997). The most widely used regimens rely on the antiprogestogen, mifepristone, which binds to progesterone receptors, inhibiting the action of progesterone and hence interfering with the continuation of pregnancy. Treatment regimens entail an initial dose of mifepristone followed by administration of a synthetic prostaglandin analogue, which enhances uterine contractions and helps expel the products of conception (Swahn and Bygdeman 1988).

The effects of medical methods of abortion are similar to those associated with spontaneous abortion and include cramping and prolonged menstrual-like bleeding. Bleeding occurs for nine days on average but can last up to 45 days in rare cases (Creinin and Aubény 1999). Side-effects include nausea, vomiting and diarrhoea. Conditions that warrant caution with the use of mifepristone and a prostaglandin include chronic or acute adrenal or hepatic failure, bleeding disorders, heavy smoking and allergies to any of the drugs used. Mifepristone is not an effective treatment for ectopic pregnancy; suspicion of ectopic pregnancy demands further investigation and, if confirmed, immediate treatment (see World Health Organization 2000a for specifics on treatment).

Medical methods of abortion have proved acceptable in several low-resource settings (Elul et al. 1999, Ngoc et al. 1999). However, the drugs, mifepristone in particular, are currently available in only a few developing countries. This may change in coming years, and programme managers should be aware of what would be required to introduce medical methods of abortion into health services.

Table 2.2 **Commonly used mifepristone plus prostaglandin regimens**

Up to 9 completed weeks since LMP	After 12 completed weeks since LMP
200 mg mifepristone followed after 36-48 hours by	200 mg mifepristone followed after 36-48 hours by
1.0 mg vaginal gemeprost	1 mg vaginal gemeprost (repeated every 6 hours up to maximum of 4 doses, and if necessary every 3 hours up to 4 additional doses)
or	
800 µg vaginal misoprostol	*or*
or	400 µg misoprostol orally every 3 hours up to 5 doses
400 µg oral misoprostol up to 7 completed weeks	*or*
	800 µg vaginal misoprostol followed by 400 µg oral misoprostol every 3 hours up to a maximum of 4 doses
	µg = micrograms
	mg = milligrams

2.4.1   Mifepristone and prostaglandin

2.4.1.1 *Up to 9 completed weeks since last menstrual period*

Mifepristone with misoprostol or gemeprost has been proved to be highly effective, safe and acceptable for early first trimester abortions (RCOG 2000). Efficacy rates up to 98% are reported (Trussell and Ellertson 1999). Approximately 2 to 5% of women treated with the mifepristone and misoprostol regimen will require surgical intervention to resolve an incomplete abortion, terminate a continuing pregnancy, or control bleeding

(World Health Organization Task Force on Post-ovulatory Methods of Fertility Regulation 2000).

The original protocols for the use of mifepristone recommended an oral dose of 600mg mifepristone followed by 1mg of vaginal gemeprost after 36-48 hours. However, several studies have established that 200mg of mifepristone is the dosage of choice since it is as effective as 600mg (McKinley et al. 1993; World Health Organization Task Force on Post-ovulatory Methods of Fertility Regulation 1993), and reduces costs.

Misoprostol, a prostaglandin which has also been shown to be effective (RCOG 2000), is considerably cheaper than gemeprost, and does not require refrigeration. It is therefore the prostaglandin of choice for most countries. An oral dose of 200mg mifepristone followed by 800 µg misoprostol administered vaginally is an effective regimen (RCOG 2000). Vaginal misoprostol has been shown to be more effective and better tolerated than misoprostol given orally (El-Refaey et al. 1995). An oral dose of 400 µg of misoprostol is effective up to 7 completed weeks of pregnancy (World Health Organization Task Force on Post-ovulatory Methods of Fertility Regulation 2000).

Most protocols require that women take both mifepristone and prostaglandin under clinical supervision, involving a second visit to the health care facility two days after receiving mifepristone to take the prostaglandin. Women may leave the facility shortly after taking the mifepristone, after being told to expect bleeding and possible expulsion of products of conception, how to recognize complications and whom to contact if they should occur. Staff should be available on a 24-hour basis to respond to such situations.

Following administration of the prostaglandin at the second visit, the standard observation period is 4-6 hours, during which up to 90% of women will expel the products of conception. Some women may require medication for cramps during this period (see 2.2.1 above). The approximately 10% of women who do not abort during the observation period should return to the health care facility about 2 weeks later to confirm that the abortion has been completed.

Protocols which allow the woman to leave the facility immediately after prostaglandin administration, call for explanation that she is likely to expel the products of conception at home or somewhere else without medical supervision. In this case, women should return to the health care facility about two weeks later to confirm completion of the abortion through a physical examination or laboratory test.

Some investigators consider that the second visit to the facility for the prostaglandin is unnecessary and suggest that women be allowed to take the prostaglandin at home (Schaff et al. 1997). This approach has recently also been used in communities in Tunisia and Viet Nam and found to be acceptable to many women (Elul et al. 2001). However, the safety and appropriateness of this approach in different settings is still the subject of review.

In the case of an incomplete or failed abortion, surgical abortion is required. Every facility offering medical methods of abortion must be able to ensure provision of vacuum aspiration in case the need arises. Such provision can be available on site or through an arrangement with another facility that performs vacuum aspiration. In all cases, health care providers must ensure that the woman can reach such services in case of an emergency.

Women are more likely to be satisfied with the procedure if they have realistic expectations (Breitbart 2000). Hence, they need complete information about what is to be expected with, and the possible side-effects of, medical methods of abortion. Health workers should ensure that women understand the importance of complying with the protocol, especially if any of the drugs are self-administered, and that they know how to recognize, and what to do in case of, complications.

2.4.1.2 *From 9 to 12 completed weeks since last menstrual period*

Mifepristone and misoprostol are also being investigated between 9 and 13 weeks of pregnancy (Ashok et al. 1998b). Initial positive findings need to be confirmed in order to establish the optimal regimens.

2.4.1.3 *After 12 completed weeks since last menstrual period*

A regimen of oral mifepristone followed by repeated doses of misoprostol or gemeprost is safe and highly effective (RCOG 2000). An oral dose of 200mg mifepristone followed by 800µg misoprostol administered vaginally 36-48 hours later and further 400µg oral doses of misoprostol every three hours, to a maximum of four doses, has been found to be effective in 97% of cases (El-Refaey and Templeton 1995). An oral dose of 400µg of misoprostol every 3 hours up to 5 doses after 200mg mifepristone has also been used successfully (Ngai et al. 2000). A vaginally administered dose of 1 mg gemeprost used after 200mg mifepristone and repeated if necessary every 6 hours up to four doses can also be used effectively (Ho et al. 1996). The treatment with gemeprost could continue with 1mg gemeprost every 3 hours for 4 additional doses if necessary (Gemzell-Danielsson and Ostlund 2000, Tang et al. 2001).

2.4.2   Misoprostol or gemeprost alone

2.4.2.1 *Up to 12 completed weeks since last menstrual period*

Misoprostol alone has also been studied in terms of effectiveness and safety. Although no comparative studies have been conducted, available data suggest that the effectiveness of misoprostol alone is lower, the procedure lasts longer and is more painful with greater gastro-intestinal side-effects than the combined regimen with mifepristone (Bugalho et al. 2000).

Because of the drug's wide availability and low cost and since in some settings its broader use has been reported to contribute to the decrease in the complications from unsafe abortion (Costa and Vessy 1993), the development of an optimal treatment regimen for the delivery of misoprostol alone is currently under investigation (Blanchard et al. 2000).

There are concerns about the consequences of ongoing pregnancies with the use of misoprostol alone (Fonseca et al. 1991, Gonzalez et al. 1998, Schonhofer 1991, Orioli and Castilla 2000). Further research is needed to evaluate the possible teratogenicity of misoprostol.

2.4.2.2 After 12 completed weeks since last menstrual period

Misoprostol has been found to be up to 84% effective in inducing abortion within 24 hours with a variety of doses administered orally or vaginally (Dickinson et al. 1998, Wong et al. 1996), although it is not as rapid as when used in combination with mifepristone. Further research is needed to identify the optimal regimen for the use of misoprostol alone for pregnancies of more than 12 weeks.

Vaginal administration of gemeprost alone is registered for termination of second-trimester pregnancy in several countries. The recommended dose is 1mg which is given every 3 hours up to 5 times during the first day and repeated the next day if necessary. With this treatment, 80% and 95% of women will abort within 24 and 48 hours, respectively (Thong et al. 1992).

2.4.3 Other medical abortion agents

Methotrexate, which is a cytotoxic drug used to treat cancer, rheumatoid arthritis, psoriasis and some other conditions, has been used in combination with misoprostol as a medical method for early abortion (up to 7 completed weeks since LMP) in some countries where mifepristone has not been available. A recent randomized controlled trial reported an overall 92% success rate with 50mg of methotrexate followed by 800µg intravaginally administered misoprostol 6 or 7 days later. Success rate at day 15 was 83% (Creinin 2000). However, a WHO Toxicology Panel recommended against the use of methotrexate for inducing abortion, based on concerns about teratogenicity (UNDP/UNFPA/WHO/World Bank Special Programme of Research, Development and Research Training in Human Reproduction 1997). Although the actual risks are yet unknown, limb defects and skull and facial abnormalities in pregnancies that continued after failed attempts to induce abortion with methotrexate have been reported (Powell and Ekert 1971, Diniz et al. 1978, Feldkamp and Carey 1993). It is therefore recommended that services that wish to introduce medical methods of abortion use mifepristone and misoprostol, not methotrexate.

Other agents are used to stimulate uterine contractions and induce abortion from 12 completed weeks since last menstrual period. They include intra-amniotic injection of hypertonic saline or hyperosmolar urea; intra- or extra-amniotic administration of ethacridine; parenteral, intra-amniotic or extra-amniotic administration of prostaglandin analogues; and intravenous or intramuscular administration of oxytocin (World Health Organization 1997). Most of these methods and routes of administration, however, are invasive and less safe than the newer medical methods.

2.5 OTHER ISSUES RELATED TO ABORTION PROCEDURES

2.5.1 Infection prevention and control

Since abortion procedures and care involve contact with blood and other body fluids, all clinical and support staff in all facilities that provide these services should understand and apply universal precautions for infection prevention and control, for both their own and their patients' protection.

Universal precautions are simple standards of infection control practices to be used in the care of all patients, at all times, to reduce the risk of transmission of bloodborne infections. They include: handwashing with soap and water before and after all procedures; use of protective barriers such as gloves, gowns, aprons, masks, goggles for direct contact with blood and other body fluids; safe disposal of waste contaminated with blood or other body fluids; proper handling of soiled linen; careful handling and disposal of "sharps"; and proper disinfection of instruments and other contaminated equipment (World Health Organization 2001).

2.5.1.1 Handwashing and use of protective barriers

All staff should wash their hands thoroughly before coming into contact with the woman and immediately after any contact with blood, body fluids or mucous membranes. High-level disinfected or sterile gloves should be worn and replaced between contacts with different clients and between vaginal (or rectal) examinations of the same woman. It should be noted that use of auxiliary supplies such as sterile booties does not make a significant difference in infection rates while it increases costs.

2.5.1.2 Cleaning

Detergents and hot water are adequate for the routine cleaning of floors, beds, toilets, walls, and rubber draw sheets. Following a spillage of body fluids, heavy-duty rubber gloves should be worn and as much body fluid as possible removed with an absorbent material. This can then be discarded in a leakproof container and later incinerated or buried in a deep pit. The area of spillage should be cleaned with a chlorine-based disinfectant and then thoroughly washed with hot soap and water.

All soiled linen should be handled as little as possible, bagged at the point of collection and not sorted or rinsed in patient care areas. If possible, linen with large amounts of body fluid should be transported in leakproof bags. If leakproof bags are not available, the linen should be folded with the soiled parts inside and handled carefully, with gloves.

2.5.1.3 Safe disposal of waste contaminated with body fluids

Solid waste that is contaminated with blood, body fluids, laboratory specimens or body tissue should be placed in leakproof containers and incinerated, or buried in a 7 foot deep pit, at least 30 feet away from a water source. Liquid waste such as blood or body fluid should be poured down a drain connected to an adequately-treated sewer or pit latrine.

2.5.1.4 Safe handling and disposal of "sharps"

The greatest hazard of HIV transmission in health care settings is through skin puncture with contaminated needles or "sharps". This also applies to hepatitis-B. Most "sharps" injuries involving such transmission are through deep injuries with hollow-bore needles. Such injuries frequently occur when needles are recapped, cleaned, disposed of, or inappropriately discarded. Although recapping needles is to be avoided whenever possible, sometimes recapping is necessary. When this is the case, a single-handed scooping method should be used. Puncture-resistant disposal containers must be available and readily accessible for the disposal of "sharps". These can be burned in a closed incinerator or buried in a deep pit. Added precautions to prevent "sharps" injuries include wearing gloves, having an adequate light source when treating women, locating "sharps" containers directly at the point of use, never discarding "sharps" in general waste, and keeping "sharps" out of the reach of children. Whenever possible, needle holders should be used when suturing.

2.5.1.5 Safe cleaning of equipment after use

Immediately after use, all reusable surgical instruments used in abortion should be sent for cleaning and sterilization. Where central services for this are not available, or in resource-poor settings, the following procedures are recommended.

The most important step to ensure proper final decontamination of instruments is physical cleaning. Instruments should immediately be washed with soap under running water. All instruments should then be sterilized or disinfected with a high-level disinfectant. Sterilization kills all microorganisms, including bacterial endospores such as those that cause tetanus and gas gangrene. It is best achieved with pressurized steam [20 minutes at 121°C and 103.5-140kPa pressure] or gas (ethylene oxide) (Sopwith et al. 2001).

High-level disinfection should be achieved by soaking instruments in a solution of hypochlorite bleach [5 minutes contact at 20-25°C with buffered hypochlorite (pH = 7-8) at a concentration of 5000ppm available chlorine], or fresh glutaraldehyde [5 hours contact at 20-25°C with a 2% activated alkaline formulation (pH = 7.5-9)] (Sopwith et al. 2001). High-level disinfection destroys all microorganisms including hepatitis-B virus and HIV but does not reliably kill bacterial endospores. The use of phenol or antiseptics will not achieve high-level disinfection. Instruments must be rinsed with *sterile* water after disinfection.

Plastic instruments, such as most vacuum aspiration syringes and cannulae currently available, cannot be exposed to high heat for sterilization, since they will crack and melt. Unless there are specific instructions to the contrary, the cold methods of high-level disinfection described above should be used.

Health workers should always refer to the instructions for use of all items being disinfected to ensure they are using the appropriate form of disinfection.

2   Methods of abortion continued

2.5.2   Managing abortion complications

When abortion is performed by appropriately trained personnel, complications are rare. Nevertheless, every service delivery site at every level of the health system should be equipped and have personnel trained to recognize abortion complications and to provide or refer women for prompt care, 24 hours a day (World Health Organization 1994). Facilities and skills required to manage abortion complications are similar to those needed to care for women who have had a miscarriage.

2.5.2.1 Incomplete abortion

Incomplete abortion is uncommon with vacuum aspiration when the abortion is performed by a skilled provider. It is more common with medical methods of abortion. Signs and symptoms include vaginal bleeding, abdominal pain and signs of infection. It should also be suspected if, upon visual examination, the tissue aspirated during surgical abortion does not conform to estimated duration of pregnancy. Staff at every health care facility should be trained and equipped to treat incomplete abortion by re-evacuating the uterus with vacuum aspiration, paying attention to the possibility of haemorrhage or infection.

2.5.2.2 Failed abortion

Failed abortion can occur in women who have undergone either surgical or medical methods of abortion. If, at the follow-up visit after either type of procedure, the pregnancy is continuing, termination of the pregnancy requires vacuum aspiration, or D&E for second-trimester pregnancies.

2.5.2.3 Haemorrhage

Haemorrhage can result from retained products of conception, trauma or damage to the cervix or, rarely, uterine perforation. Depending on the cause, appropriate treatment may include re-evacuation of the uterus and administration of uterotonic drugs to stop the bleeding, intravenous fluid replacement, and, in severe cases, blood transfusion, laparoscopy or exploratory laparotomy. Because of the low incidence of haemorrhage using vacuum aspiration, it is not recommended to use oxytocics routinely, although they may be required with D&E. Prolonged menstrual-like bleeding is an expected effect of medical methods of abortion. Such bleeding rarely is heavy enough to constitute an emergency. However, every service-delivery site must be able to stabilize and treat or refer women with haemorrhage as quickly as possible.

2.5.2.4 Infection

Infection rarely occurs following properly performed abortion. Common symptoms include fever or chills, foul-smelling vaginal or cervical discharge, abdominal or pelvic pain, prolonged vaginal bleeding or spotting, uterine tenderness, and/or an elevated white blood cell count. When infection is diagnosed, health care staff should administer antibiotics and, if retained products of conception are a likely cause of infection, re-evacuate the uterus. Women with severe infections may require hospitalization. As discussed in section 1.6 above, prophylactic prescription of antibiotics for women undergoing surgical abortion has been found to reduce the risk of post-abortion infection (Sawaya et al. 1996) and should be provided where possible.

2.5.2.5 Uterine perforation

Usually, uterine perforation goes undetected and resolves without the need for intervention. A study of more than 700 women undergoing concurrent first-trimester abortion and laparoscopic sterilization found that 12 out of the 14 uterine perforations were so small that they would not have been recognized had laparoscopy not been performed (Kaali et al. 1989). Where uterine perforation is suspected, observation and antibiotics may be all that is necessary. Where available, laparoscopy is the investigative method of choice. If the laparoscopy examination and/or the status of the patient gives rise to any suspicion of damage to bowel, blood vessels or other structures, a laparotomy to repair damaged tissues may be needed.

2.5.2.6 Anaesthesia-related complications

Local anaesthesia is safer than general anaesthesia, both for vacuum aspiration in the first trimester and for dilatation and evacuation in the second trimester (Osborn et al. 1990, MacKay et al. 1985). Where general anaesthesia is used, staff must be skilled in stabilization management of convulsions and impairment of cardiorespiratory function. Narcotic reversal agents should always be readily available.

2.5.2.7 Long-term sequelae

The vast majority of women who have a properly performed induced abortion will not suffer any long-term effects on their general or reproductive health. The exceptions are a proportion of the small number of women who have severe complications of abortion (World Health Organization 1997).

Research shows no association between safely induced first-trimester abortion and adverse outcomes of subsequent pregnancies (Hogue et al. 1999). Sound epidemiological data show no increased risk of breast cancer for women undergoing first-trimester abortion (Melbye et al. 1997). According to a comprehensive review (Dagg 1991), adverse psychological sequelae occur in a very small number of women and appear to be the continuation of pre-existing conditions.

3 Follow-up

3.1 RECOVERY PERIOD

3.1.1 Surgical methods of abortion

During the observation period following abortion performed by surgical means, staff should offer women comfort and support and monitor their recovery. Health workers should take special note of women's reports of pain, since pain may be due to uterine perforation or acute haematometra – blood filling the uterus – which can be treated by inducing uterine contractions with ergometric drugs. Thus, particularly with late abortions, it is important to confirm the size of the uterus through the abdominal wall bimanually. In the absence of complications, most women can leave the health care facility as soon as they feel able and their vital signs are normal. After abortions performed later in pregnancy and after heavy sedation or general anaesthesia, recovery periods may be longer and women may require closer observation.

Ideally, women undergoing surgical abortion should have a follow-up visit with a trained practitioner 7-10 days after the procedure, to assess general health.

3.1.2 Medical methods of abortion

As described earlier, treatment protocols for medical methods of abortion used up to 9 completed weeks of pregnancy generally require women to remain under clinical observation for 4-6 hours after taking the prostaglandin. Providers should inspect all sanitary pads and bed pans used during the period of observation, maximizing the opportunity to confirm an abortion during this time.

Women for whom complete abortion is not confirmed at that time, those who take the prostaglandin at home or those who leave the facility shortly after prostaglandin administration should be scheduled for a return visit in 10-15 days to confirm that the abortion has been completed, that there is no infection, and that no other complications have occurred. In most cases, complete abortion will be confirmed at this visit. If not, women may opt to undergo vacuum aspiration, but it is not clinically necessary for them to do so unless the physical examination, the clinical symptoms or a laboratory test suggest that the pregnancy is still growing.

In view of the greater risk of haemorrhage and of incomplete abortion associated with procedures undertaken after 12 completed weeks of pregnancy, all women in these cases should remain under observation until both fetus and placenta have been expelled.

3.2 CONTRACEPTIVE METHOD PROVISION AND STI COUNSELLING

Staff should ensure that women receive information and counselling on post-abortion contraception, including emergency contraception, before they leave the health care facility.

All methods of contraception, including intrauterine devices and hormonal contraceptives, can be considered for use after abortion, as long as attention is paid to each woman's health profile and the limitations associated with certain methods (see Annex 4). The diaphragm and cervical cap should not be used until about 6 weeks after a second-trimester abortion and there is a higher risk of expulsion of intrauterine devices if inserted at the time of a second-trimester abortion (Stanwood et al. 2001). Some natural family planning methods should only be started three cycles after an abortion (World Health Organization 2000b). Special attention should be given in cases where women request sterilization to ensure their choice is not influenced by the crisis nature of the moment and to avoid later regret.

Abortion service delivery sites should be able to provide most methods in the facility if the woman chooses a method. If the contraceptive chosen by the woman cannot be provided (e.g. sterilization is rarely offered at primary care level), the woman should be given information about where and how she can get it and offered an interim method. All women should be informed about emergency contraception and consideration should be given to providing it to women who choose not to start using a routine contraceptive method immediately.

Providers should discuss prevention of STIs including HIV and the importance of condom use with all women regardless of the contraceptive method chosen. Information about infection prevention should be particularly emphasized for people who may be at increased risk, and in areas of known high prevalence of HIV. Voluntary testing and counselling may be offered, or referral to HIV counselling and testing in other facilities. Dual protection, or the use of methods to protect against both pregnancy and STIs, should be promoted.

3.3 INSTRUCTIONS FOR CARE AFTER ABORTION

Women undergoing abortion should receive clear, simple, oral and written instructions about how to care for themselves after leaving the health care facility, including how to recognize complications that require medical attention. While they wait for a medically induced abortion to be completed, women should be able to contact a physician or other health worker who can answer questions and provide support.

3　Follow-up *continued*

After a surgical abortion, women may experience light menstrual-like bleeding or spotting for several weeks. Women should be informed that bleeding similar to or heavier than a heavy menstrual period might be expected with medical methods of abortion. Symptoms that warrant clinical attention include excessive bleeding, fever lasting more than one day and pelvic pain. Nausea, sometimes accompanied by vomiting, generally subsides within 24 hours after abortion performed by surgical methods. Staff should advise women to expect cramping, which they can usually alleviate sufficiently with non-prescription analgesics. Information on recognizing complications and how to seek help for them should be made available in pictorial form for women who cannot read.

After first-trimester abortion, most women can return to their usual activities and responsibilities within hours or days.

The follow-up visit is an opportunity for providers to talk with women about their experiences, if needed. For instance, women having an abortion for medical reasons or following rape may need to speak about their sense of loss or ambivalence, or may want additional counselling.

References

Ashok PW, Penney GC, Flett GMM and Templeton A. (1998a) An effective regimen for early medical abortion: a report of 2000 consecutive cases. *Human Reproduction* 13:2962-2965.

Ashok PW, Flett GM and Templeton A. (1998b) Termination of pregnancy at 9-13 weeks' amenorrhoea with mifepristone and misoprostol. Lancet 352:542-543.

Blanchard K, Winikoff B, Coyaji K and Ngoc NTN. (2000) Misoprostol alone: a new method of medical abortion? *Journal of the American Medical Women's Association* 55:189-190.

Borgatta L and Nickinovich D. (1997) Pain during early abortion. *Journal of Reproductive Medicine* 42:287-293.

Breitbart V. (2000) Counseling for medical abortion. *American Journal of Obstetrics and Gynecology* 183(Suppl 2):S26-S33.

Bugalho A, Mocumbi S, Faúndes A and David E. (2000) Termination of pregnancies <6 weeks gestation with a single dose of 800 µg of vaginal misoprostol. *Contraception* 61:47-50.

Cade L and Ashley J. (1993) Prophylactic paracetamol for analgesia after vaginal termination of pregnancy. *Anaesthesia & Intensive Care* 21:93-96.

Cameron IT and Baird DT. (1988) The return to ovulation following early abortion: a comparison between vacuum aspiration and prostaglandin. *Acta Endocrinologica (Copenhagen)* 118:161-167.

Cates W, Grimes DA and Schultz KF. (2000) Abortion surveillance at CDC : creating public health light out of political heat. *American Journal of Preventive Medicine* 19(Suppl 1):12-17.

Costa SH and Vessy MP. (1993) Misoprostol and illegal abortion in Rio de Janeiro, Brazil. *Lancet* 341:1258-1261.

Creinin MD. (2000) Randomized comparison of efficacy, acceptability and cost of medical versus surgical abortion. *Contraception* 62:117-124.

Creinin MD and Aubény E. (1999) Medical abortion in early pregnancy. In Paul M, Lichtenberg ES, Borgatta L, Grimes D and Stubblefield PG (eds). *A clinician's guide to medical and surgical abortion.* New York, Churchill Livingstone, pp. 91-106.

Dagg PKB. (1991) The psychological sequelae of therapeutic abortion – denied and completed. *American Journal of Psychiatry* 148:578-585.

Dahl V, Fjellanger F and Raeder JC. (2000) No effect of preoperative paracetamol and codeine suppositories for pain after termination of pregnancies in general anaesthesia. *European Journal of Pain* 4:211-215.

Dickinson JE, Godfrey M and Evans SF. (1998) Efficacy of intravaginal misoprostol in second-trimester pregnancy termination: a randomized controlled trial. *Journal of Maternal-Fetal Medicine* 7:115-119.

Diniz EM, Corradini HB, Ramos JL and Brock R. (1978) Efietos sobre o concepto do metotrexato (ametopterina) administrado à mãe. Apresentação de caso. *Revista do Hospital das Clinicas; Faculdade de Medicine a Universidade de Sao Paulo* 33:286-290.

Donati S, Medda E, Proietti S, Rizzo L, Spinelli A, Subrizi D and Grandolfo ME. (1996) Reducing pain of first trimester abortion under local anaesthesia. *European Journal of Obstetrics & Gynecology and Reproductive Biology* 70:145-149.

El-Refaey H and Templeton A. (1995) Induction of abortion in the second trimester by a combination of misoprostol and mifepristone: a randomized comparison between two misoprostol regimens. *Human Reproduction* 10:475-478.

El-Refaey H, Rajasekar D, Abdalla M, Calder L and Templeton A. (1995) Induction of abortion with mifepristone (RU486) and oral or vaginal misoprostol. *New England Journal of Medicine* 382:983-987.

Elul B, Ellertson C, Winikoff B and Coyaji K. (1999) Side effects of mifepristone-misoprostol abortion versus surgical abortion. Data from a trial in China, Cuba and India. *Contraception* 59:107-114.

Elul B, Hajri S, Ngoc NN, Ellertson C, Slama CB, Pearlman E and Winikoff B. (2001) Can women in less-developed countries use a simplified medical abortion regimen? *Lancet* 357:1402-1405.

Feldkamp M and Carey JC. (1993) Clinical teratology counseling and consultation case report: low dose methotrexate exposure in the early weeks of pregnancy. *Teratology* 47:533-539.

Finn R, Clarke CA, Donohoe WTA, McConnell RB, Sheppard PM, Lehane D and Kulke W. (1961) Experimental studies on the prevention of Rh haemolytic disease. *British Medical Journal* 1:1486-1490.

Fonseca W, Alencar AJ, Mota FS and Coelho HL. (1991) Misoprostol and congenital malformations. *Lancet* 338:56.

Gemzell-Danielsson K and Ostlund E. (2000) Termination of second trimester pregnancy with mifepristone and gemeprost. The clinical experience of 197 consecutive cases. *Acta Obstetricia et Gynecologica Scandinavica* 79:702-706.

References *continued*

Gonzalez CH, Marques-Dias MJ, Kim CA, Sugayama SM, Da Pa JA, Huson SM and Holmes LB. (1998) Congenital abnormalities in Brazilian children associated with misoprostol misuse in first trimester of pregnancy. *Lancet* 351:1624-1627.

Greenslade FC, Benson J, Winkler J, Henderson V, Wolf M and Leonard A. (1993) Summary of clinical and programmatic experience with manual vacuum aspiration. *IPAS Advances in Abortion Care* 3(2):1-4.

Grimes DA and Cates W Jr. (1979) Complications from legally-induced abortion: a review. *Obstetrical and Gynecological Survey* 34:177-191.

Grimes DA, Hulka JF and McCutchen ME. (1980) Midtrimester abortion by dilatation and evacuation versus intra-amniotic instillation of prostaglanding F2 alpha: a randomized clinical trial. *American Journal of Obstetrics and Gynecology* 137:785-790.

Grimes D, Schulz KF, Cates W and Tyler CW. (1977) The Joint Program for the Study of Abortion/CDC – a preliminary report. In Hern W and Andrikopolous B (eds). *Abortion in the seventies.* New York, National Abortion Federation, pp. 41-46.

Grimes DA, Schulz KF and Cates W Jr. (1984) Prevention of uterine perforation during currettage abortion. *JAMA* 251:2108-2112.

Hakim-Elahi E, Tovell HM and Burnhill MS. (1990) Complications of first trimester abortion: a report of 170,000 cases. *Obstetrics & Gynecology* 76:129-135.

Hein A, Jakobsson J and Ryberg G. (1999) Paracetamol 1 g given rectally at the end of minor gynaecological surgery is not efficacious in reducing postoperative pain. *Acta Anaesthesiologia Scandinavica* 43:245-247.

Henshaw RC and Templeton AA. (1991) Pre-operative cervical preparation before first trimester vacuum aspiration: a randomized controlled comparison between gemeprost and mifepristone (RU 486). *British Journal of Obstetrics and Gynaecology* 98:1025-1030.

Ho PC, Chan YF and Lau W. (1996) Misoprostol is as effective as gemeprost in termination of second trimester pregnancy when combined with mifepristone: a randomised comparative trial. *Contraception* 53:281-283.

Hogue CJ, Boardman LA, Stotland NL and Peipert JF. (1999) Answering questions about long-term outcomes. In Paul M, Lichtenberg ES, Borgatta L, Grimes D and Stubblefield PG (eds). *A clinician's guide to medical and surgical abortion.* Philadelphia, Churchill Livingstone, pp 217-228.

Kaali SG, Szigetvari IA and Bartfai GS. (1989) The frequency and management of uterine perforations during first-trimester abortions. *American Journal of Obstetrics and Gynecology* 161:406-408.

Lawson HW, Frye A, Atrash HK, Smith JC, Shulman HB and Ramick M. (1994) Abortion mortality, United States, 1972 through 1987. *American Journal of Obstetrics and Gynecology* 171:1365-1372.

Lean TH, Vengadasalam D, Pachauri S and Miller ER. (1976) A comparison of D&C and vacuum aspiration for performing first trimester abortion. *International Journal of Gynecology & Obstetrics* 14:481-486.

MacKay HT, Schulz KF and Grimes DA. (1985) Safety of local versus general anaesthesia for second trimester dilatation and evacuation abortion. *Obstetrics and Gynecology* 66:661-665.

Matambo J, Moodley J and Chigumadzi P. (1999) Analgesia for termination of pregnancy. *South African Medical Journal* 89:816.

McKinley C, Thong KJ and Baird DT. (1993) The effect of dose of mifepristone and gestation on the efficacy of medical abortion with mifepristone and misoprostol. *Human Reproduction* 8:1502-1505.

Melbye M, Wohlfahrt J, Olsen JH, Frisch M, Westergaard T, Helweg-Larsen K and Andersen PK. (1997) Induced abortion and the risk of breast cancer. *New England Journal of Medicine* 336:81-85.

Ngai SW, Chan YM, Tang OS and Ho PC. (1999) The use of misoprostol for pre-operative cervical dilatation prior to vacuum aspiration: a randomized trial. *Human Reproduction* 8:2139-2142.

Ngai SW, Tang OS and Ho PC. (2000) Randomized comparison of vaginal (200 microg every 3 h) and oral (400 microg every 3h) misoprostol when combined with mifepristone in termination of second trimester pregnancy. *Human Reproduction* 15:2205-2208.

Ngoc NN, Winikoff B, Clark S, Ellertson C, Am KN, Hieu DT and Elul B. (1999) Safety, efficacy and acceptability of mifepristone-misoprostol medical abortion in Vietnam. *International Family Planning Perspectives* 25:10-14 & 33.

Orioli IM and Castilla EE. (2000) Epidemiological assessment of misoprostol teratogenicity. *British Journal of Obstetrics and Gynaecology* 107:519-523.

Osborn JF, Arisi E, Spinelli A and Stazi MA. (1990) General anaesthesia, a risk factor for complication following induced abortion? *European Journal of Epidemiology* 6:416-422.

Penney GC, Thomson M, Norman J, McKenzie H, Vale L, Smith R and Imrie M. (1998) A randomised comparison of strategies for reducing infective complications of induced abortion. *British Journal of Obstetrics and Gynaecology* 105:599-604.

Peyron R, Aubény E, Targosz V, Silvestre L, Renault M, Elkik F, Leclerc P, Ulmann A and Baulieu EE. (1993) Early termination of pregnancy with mifepristone (RU486) and the orally active prostaglandin misoprostol. *New England Journal of Medicine* 21:1509-1513.

Powell HR and Ekert H. (1971) Methotrexate-induced congenital malformations. *Medical Journal of Australia* 2:1076-1077.

RCOG – Royal College of Obstetricians and Gynaecologists. (2000) *The care of women requesting induced abortion.* Evidence-based guideline No.7. London, RCOG Press.

Sawaya GF, Grady D, Kerlikowske K and Grimes DA. (1996) Antibiotics at the time of induced abortion: the case for universal prophylaxis based on a meta-analysis. *Obstetrics and Gynecology* 87:884-890.

Schaff EA, Eisinger SH, Stadalius LS, Franks P, Gore BZ and Popperna S. (1999) Low-dose mifepristone 200mg and vaginal misoprostol for abortion. *Contraception* 59:1-6.

Schaff EA, Stadalius LS, Eisinger SH and Franks P. (1997) Vaginal misoprostol administered at home after mifepristone (RU486) for abortion. *Journal of Family Practice* 44:353-360.

Schonhofer PS. (1991) Brazil: misuse of misoprostol as an abortifacient may induce malformations. *Lancet* 337:1534-1535.

Schulz KF, Grimes DA and Cates W Jr. (1983) Measures to prevent cervical injury during suction curettage abortion. *Lancet* 1:1182-1184.

Singh K, Fong YF, Prasad RNV and Dong F. (1998) Randomized trial to determine optimal dose of vaginal misoprostol for preabortion cervical priming. *Obstetrics and Gynecology* 92:795-798.

References *continued*

Smith GM, Stubblefield PG, Chirchirillo L and McCarthy MJ. (1979) Pain of first trimester abortion: its quantification and relations with other variables. *American Journal of Obstetrics and Gynecology* 133:489-498.

Solo J. (2000) Easing the pain: pain management in the treatment of incomplete abortion. *Reproductive Health Matters* 8:45-51.

Sopwith W, Garner P, Hart A. (2001) Preventing infection from reusable medical equipment: a systematic review of decontamination procedures. *Liverpool School of Tropical Medicine.* Available online at: www.liv.ac.uk/lstm/deconreview.html.

Spitz IM, Bardin CW, Benton L and Robbins A. (1998) Early pregnancy termination with mifepristone and misoprostol in the United States. *New England Journal of Medicine* 338:1241-1247.

Stanwood NL, Grimes DA and Schulz KF. (2001) Insertion of an intrauterine contraceptive device after induced or spontaneous abortion: a review of the evidence. *British Journal of Obstetrics and Gynaecology* 108:1168-1173.

Suprapto K and Reed S. (1984) Naproxen sodium for pain relief in first-trimester abortion. *American Journal of Obstetrics and Gynecology* 150:1000-1001.

Swahn ML and Bygdeman M. (1988) The effect of the antiprogestin RU486 on uterine contractility and sensitivity to prostaglandin and oxytocin. *British Journal of Obstetrics and Gynaecology* 95:126-134.

Tang OS, Thong KJ and Baird DT. (2001) Second trimester medical abortion with mifepristone and gemeprost: a review of 956 cases. *Contraception* 64:29-32.

Thong KJ, Robertson AJ and Baird DT. (1992) A retrospective study of 932 second trimester terminations using gemeprost (16, 16 dimethyl-trans delta 2 PGE1 methyl ester). *Prostaglandins* 44:65-74.

Thonneau P, Fougeyrollas B, Ducot B, Boubilley D, Dif J, Lalande M and Soulat C. (1998) Complications of abortion performed under local anesthesia. *European Journal of Obstetrics & Gynaecology and Reproductive Biology* 81:59-63.

Trussell J and Ellertson C. (1999) Estimating the efficacy of medical abortion. *Contraception* 60:119-135.

UNDP/UNFPA/WHO/World Bank Special Programme of Research, Development and Research Training in Human Reproduction. (1997) Methotrexate for the termination of early pregnancy: a toxicology review. *Reproductive Health Matters* 9: 162-166.

Urquhart DR and Templeton AA. (1990) Reduced risk of isoimmunisation in medical abortion. *Lancet* 335:914.

Urquhart DR, Templeton AA, Shinewi F, Chapman M, Hawkins K, McGarry J, Rodger M, Baird DT et al. (1997) The efficacy and tolerance of mifepristone and prostaglandin in termination of pregnancy of less than 63 days gestation; UK multicentre study – final results. *Contraception* 55:1-5.

Westfall JM, O'Brien-Gonzales A and Barley G. (1998) Update on early medical and surgical abortion. *Journal of Women's Health* 7:991-995.

Winikoff B, Sivin I, Coyaji KJ, Cabezas E, Xiao B, Gu S, Du MK, Krishna UR, Eschen A and Ellertson C. (1997) Safety, efficacy, and acceptability of medical abortion in China, Cuba and India: a comparative trial of mifepristone-misoprostol versus surgical abortion. *American Journal of Obstetrics and Gynecology* 176:431-437.

Wong KS, Ngai CSW, Khan KS, Tang LC and Ho PC. (1996) Termination of second trimester pregnancy with gemeprost and misoprostol: a randomized double-blind placebo-controlled trial. *Contraception* 54:23-25.

World Health Organization. (1994) *Clinical management of abortion complications: a practical guide.* Geneva, World Health Organization. (WHO/FHE/MSM/94.1)

World Health Organization. (1997) *Medical methods for termination of pregnancy.* WHO Technical Report Series 871. Geneva, World Health Organization.

World Health Organization. (1999) *HIV and pregnancy: a review.* Geneva, World Health Organization. (WHO/CHS/RHR/99.15)

World Health Organization. (2000a) *Managing the complications of pregnancy and childbirth: a guide for midwives and doctors.* Geneva, World Health Organization. (WHO/RHR/00.7)

World Health Organization. (2000b) *Improving access to quality care in family planning: medical eligibility criteria for contraceptive methods.* Second edition. Geneva, World Health Organization. (WHO/RHR/00.02)

World Health Organization. (2001) *Fact Sheet 11: HIV and the workplace and universal precautions.* Geneva, World Health Organization. Available online at: www.who.int/HIV_AIDS/nursemidwives/fact-sheet-11.

World Health Organization Task Force on Post-ovulatory Methods for Fertility Regulation. (1993) Termination of pregnancy with reduced doses of mifepristone. *British Medical Journal* 307:532-537.

World Health Organization Task Force on Post-ovulatory Methods for Fertility Regulation. (1994) Cervical ripening with mifepristone (RU 486) in late first trimester abortion. *Contraception* 50:461-475.

World Health Organization Task Force on Post-ovulatory Methods for Fertility Regulation. (2000) Comparison of two doses of mifepristone in combination with misoprostol for early medical abortion: a randomised trial. *British Journal of Obstetrics and Gynaecology* 107:524-530.

Chapter **3** Putting services in place

Chapter 3 Summary

Planning and managing abortion services requires consideration of a number of factors which are applicable irrespective of the circumstances under which abortion is legal, or who has responsibility for decision-making and/or implementation within the health system. They apply whether services are public, private or non-governmental. In most cases, minor adaptations of existing facilities, acquisition of minimal additional equipment, or provision of basic training can allow for services to be provided where none previously existed or can improve the quality, safety, efficiency, and capacity, of existing services. These adaptations should be based on careful planning that encompasses the following:

- Assessment of the current situation. This need not be long or complex. Items to review in such an assessment are: laws and regulations governing availability of and access to safe abortion care; the extent and level of services currently available; the quality of services as currently provided, including the procedures being used for inducing abortion and dealing with complications of unsafe abortion; characteristics of users; and the attitudes and knowledge of health care providers.

- Establishment of national norms and standards governing the provision of quality abortion care. These norms and standards should cover: types of abortion services and where they can be provided; essential equipment, supplies, medications and facility capabilities; referral mechanisms; respect for women's informed decision-making, autonomy, confidentiality and privacy, with attention to the special needs of adolescents; and special provisions for women who have suffered rape.

- Definition of provider skills, training, supervision and certification processes. In particular, it must be clear which types of health care providers can provide abortion. Other details to be elaborated include the essential content for curricula on abortion services, supervision standards, and certification and licensing requirements to ensure that providers and institutions meet essential criteria for provision of safe abortion.

- Monitoring and evaluation of services. This includes the collection of routine service statistics and patient information, the use of supervisor checklists, and periodic special studies.

- Financing. Health service budgets should include costs of staff, training programmes, instruments, supplies and medications, and capital costs. Consideration also needs to be given to making services affordable to women who need them. Costs of adding safe abortion services to existing health services are likely to be modest, relative to the gains for women's health.

1   Assessing the current situation

Assessment will help identify where services need to be established and/or how existing services need to be improved. Basic assessment at national, regional and local levels need not be long or complex. In most cases, a review of existing information, consultation with all relevant "stakeholders" (including Ministry of Health officials, service providers, women, relevant representatives of civil society, and technical/donor agencies) and observations of service delivery at various levels of the health service, will provide the necessary information. References giving details of such approaches (rapid assessment techniques and situation analyses) are listed in Annex 1.

One methodology which has been used effectively in a variety of countries is the Strategic Approach to Improving the Quality of Care of Reproductive Health Services (World Health Organization 1999, World Health Organization 2002a). The Strategic Approach relies on the creation of an assessment team representing a broad range of stakeholders who conduct a field-based assessment of the available technologies, the quality of services being provided and women's needs and perspectives.

Whatever assessment approach is used, it is important to ensure that multiple perspectives are incorporated. This helps to ensure that recommendations and plans based on the assessment will be broadly acceptable and therefore more likely to be implemented. It is particularly important to include users' and potential users' perspectives on services as they are the main source of identifying barriers to service use. It is also important that the assessment examine people's access to reproductive health services generally, and specifically their access to contraceptive information and services, since these have an impact on the incidence of unintended pregnancy. When the assessment includes direct observation of women and providers, it is essential to obtain prior informed consent from both.

Examples of questions to answer through an assessment are listed below. The typical data sources for answering these questions will be health service records (both local and national), reports to the Ministry of Health, local or national social science studies on providers' and/or users' perspectives and, to some limited extent, the Demographic and Health Surveys (DHS) and other national health surveys. Much may be gleaned from reviewing existing literature, but in most cases such review will need to be supplemented with information from a rapid assessment. With all these sources, it is important to note that under-reporting about abortion – whether legal or illegal, safe or unsafe – is widespread.

a) What are the laws, policies and regulations, including clinic policies, governing availability of, and access to, safe abortion care?

Health professionals and the public may assume that the law is much more restrictive than it is, and thus services may not be available or women may not have the access to which they are entitled by law. Alternatively, health professionals may be aware of the law, but do not put it into practice for a variety of reasons. Close examination by both legal and public health experts of the text of the law and how the law is enacted in practice is an important step in an assessment.

- For example, where laws and policies require third party authorization or certification, such as hospital abortion committees, spousal authorization or medical or police certification of forceful intercourse, the rapid assessment will probably reveal excessive delays, causing harm to women's health. The assessment may suggest opportunities or approaches to streamline procedures and/or inform the public, lawyers, judges and doctors more clearly about when women are eligible for services and how they can access them. Effecting such change may take time, but this has been done successfully in some countries (Veira Villela and de Oliveira Araujo 2000, Billings et al. 2002).

b) What is the incidence of legal abortion and of the complications of unsafe abortion? Who is using the current services, and who is not obtaining access?

Estimating the incidence of unsafe abortion, and the numbers of legal abortions currently carried out may be difficult, especially in situations where access to legal abortion is restricted. In almost all situations, however, social science studies often furnish data which can help to establish a general picture of the situation (Mundigo and Indriso 1999). Health service statistics can provide estimates of legal abortions and numbers of hospital admissions for complications of unsafe abortion. Survey data, for instance from DHS, may exist on the extent of unwanted or ill-timed pregnancy. Where available, data on the age, marital and socio-economic status of women using legal abortion services and women suffering complications from unsafe abortions will give an indication of which women are currently using services. These data can then be used to tailor programme design.

- For example, if information about women treated for the complications of unsafe abortion reveals that they are in the under-25 age group, policy-makers and programme planners will need to develop strategies to provide young people with information and education about sexual and reproductive health, and about availability of contraceptive and abortion services. Additional information about health providers' attitudes may suggest further training for them to be open and non-judgemental with adolescents and young people.

c) Where are legal abortion services currently carried out?

Are they available at primary health care level, secondary level or only at tertiary care level? Are these public, private or non-governmental facilities? Are they provided in all parts of the country? Are they freestanding or integrated with other health services? What proportion of abortion services is provided in each of these kinds of facilities?

- The assessment may indicate that services are primarily available only in urban hospitals. In this case, the initial priority might be to train and equip staff in lower-level facilities including those in rural areas, at least to provide first-trimester procedures and effective referral for more complicated cases.

d) What is the current quality of care in abortion service delivery?

What procedures are used for inducing abortion, and for dealing with the complications of unsafe abortion, at different durations of pregnancy? What is the technical quality of these services? Is appropriate information provided to women? Do women receive pre- and post-abortion contraceptive counselling and services? Does the quality of care vary at different levels of service delivery or in different regions of the country? Some of this information may be available from health service records. A review of service protocols will indicate whether, as a matter of policy, quality of care standards are clear and whether women are to be given contraceptive information and services after abortion. Rapid assessment would determine whether practices meet the standards.

- Direct observation of services during the assessment may reveal poor quality of care such as lack of necessary supplies, failure to ensure privacy, or poor technical skills of providers. Such shortcomings can be addressed by investment in logistics systems, or improved training and supervision, for example.

e) What are the attitudes and knowledge of health care providers concerning abortion?

How knowledgeable are they about both the law and clinical techniques and about where services can be obtained? How well do their responses match practices identified by the team during rapid assessment? Existing information on these aspects is quite limited in most countries, but gathering it is important because health care providers' attitudes and practices are important determinants of women's access to safe, legal services.

- For instance, the assessment may reveal that some providers, or potential providers, feel ambivalent or negative about abortion, even where it is legal on request (Dickson-Tetteh et al. 2000). In this case, programme planners will need to consider ways to ensure that eligible women can access services.

f) What are women's knowledge about and perspectives on abortion and abortion services?

Women's knowledge and perceptions about services and the social context may also represent a barrier to using the services to which they are entitled. Studies show that women often fear mistreatment, negative attitudes of husbands or partners, or social condemnation (Mundigo and Indriso 1999), all of which inhibit their seeking care. An assessment should also determine whether women know about their rights with regard to abortion, and how much it costs to obtain an abortion in both the public and private sectors.

- For example, if the rapid assessment reveals that women dislike public services and do not use them for a variety of reasons such as lack of confidentiality/privacy, fear of criticism, or perceived poor quality of care, programme planners and managers will need to take measures to improve the quality of care. This could be addressed through refresher training for providers to update their technical and inter-personal communication skills.

g) What is the cost to the health system of providing safe abortion? What are the costs of treating the complications of unsafe abortion?

Information on direct costs may be available through health service records, or obtained through a rapid survey of health services, both public and private. More comprehensive information on costs can be obtained through more in-depth studies. Estimates for one year at one institution are adequate for the purpose of initial assessment (King et al. 1998). Information can also be analysed by applying costing spreadsheet tools (see Annex 1).

- This information will help guide rational decision-making about what services can be provided at what level of the health system, and what methods could be introduced at each level.

2 Establishing national norms and standards

In many countries, written norms and standards for abortion service delivery do not exist, and in these situations they need to be established. Where they already exist, they should be reviewed regularly to ensure standards reflect new evidence of best practice. Norms and standards should be framed to ensure that good-quality abortion services are available to the extent permitted by law. They should set criteria for providing the essential elements of good-quality abortion care delivered by public, private and non-governmental agencies, including:

- Types of abortion services and where they can be provided;

- Essential equipment, supplies, medications and facility capabilities;

- Referral mechanisms;

- Respect for women's informed decision-making, autonomy, confidentiality and privacy, with attention to the special needs of adolescents;

- Special provisions for women who have suffered rape.

2.1   TYPES OF ABORTION SERVICES AND WHERE THEY CAN BE PROVIDED

Establishing early abortion services at the primary level can greatly improve access for eligible women. Training and equipping health professionals at the primary level to provide early abortion services and to make appropriate referrals may thus be one of the most important investments to consider. Where capacity to provide quality reproductive health services at the primary level does not yet exist, a minimum step is to create effective referral mechanisms from primary to higher levels.

In all situations, a well-functioning referral system is essential (see section 2.3). Higher-level facilities, with appropriate investments in training and equipment, can be used to train health workers from lower-level facilities, thereby extending the geographic reach through the health system.

In cases where services are widespread but of poor quality, the first steps will be to assess the main reasons for the shortcomings, and develop and implement recommendations. This may include retraining staff, or improving infrastructure and equipment at all levels of the system. In most cases, integration of abortion services into existing reproductive health services is likely to be the easiest and most cost-effective strategy.

2.1.1   Community level

Community-based health workers play an important role in helping women avoid unwanted pregnancy through providing information and contraceptives, and informing them about the consequences of unsafe abortion. They also need to be able to inform women how to obtain safe, legal abortion care without undue delay, and refer women with complications of unsafe abortion for appropriate care.

2.1.2   Primary-care facility level

Primary health-care centres generally have basic medical capacity and some trained health care workers. Both vacuum aspiration and medical methods of abortion can be considered at this level, since they do not require overnight stay.

Staff are likely to include nurses, midwives, health assistants, and, in some contexts, physicians. Health personnel who have already been trained and have demonstrated ability to perform a bimanual pelvic examination to diagnose signs of pregnancy and to perform a transcervical procedure such as IUD insertion, can be trained to perform vacuum aspiration (Freedman et al. 1986, Greenslade et al. 1993). Where medical methods of abortion are registered and available, such staff can also administer and supervise the treatment (Coyaji 2000).

As with management of normal birth and of spontaneous abortion, referral arrangements must be in place to ensure prompt, higher level of care, if required. For this reason, trained staff should be available on call during and after health centre hours, in case of need.

2.1.3   District hospital (first referral) level

District hospital level facilities should offer all primary-care level abortion services as outlined in Table 3.1, even where such services are also available at lower levels of care. Specialized elements of care are rarely required for abortion and should not be a routine part of abortion service delivery, especially where resources are limited.

For example, routine use of specialized equipment such as ultrasound for early abortion increases costs to the health system and is not necessary for the provision of early abortion (RCOG 2000). General anaesthesia should not normally be used for early abortion since it increases the risks and costs of the procedure (Lawson et al. 1994). Hospitals should therefore offer abortion care on an outpatient basis, which is safe, minimizes costs and enhances convenience to the woman.

Referral hospitals that are staffed and equipped to provide emergency obstetric care are capable of managing the complications of abortion. They should therefore be prepared to accept abortion-related referrals from health care facilities throughout the catchment area.

2.1.4   Secondary and tertiary referral hospitals

Secondary and tertiary hospitals should have staff and facility capacity to perform abortions in all circumstances permitted by law and to manage all complications of unsafe abortion. The provision of abortion care at teaching hospitals is particularly important to ensure that relevant cadres of health professionals develop competence in abortion service delivery during clinical training rotations.

Table 3.1 **Types of services suitable to each level of the health care system**

Community level

- Public health education/information on reproductive health, including family planning and abortion
- Community-based distribution of appropriate methods of contraception, including emergency contraception
- All health workers trained to provide information on, and referral to, legal abortion services
- All health workers trained to recognize abortion complications and promptly refer women for treatment
- Transportation to services for abortion and for management of complications of unsafe abortion
- All health workers (and other key community professionals such as police or teachers) trained to recognize signs that girls or women have been subjected to rape or incest and to provide referral to health or other social services

Primary-care facility level

- All elements of care mentioned for the community level
- All health care workers providing reproductive health services trained to provide counselling on family planning, unwanted pregnancy and abortion
- A broader range of contraceptive methods (including, e.g., IUDs and injectables)
- Vacuum aspiration up to 12 completed weeks of pregnancy (see Chapter 2)
- Medical methods of abortion up to 9 completed weeks of pregnancy (see Chapter 2)
- Clinical stabilization of, and provision of antibiotics to, women with complications of unsafe abortion
- Vacuum aspiration for incomplete abortion
- Prompt referral and transport for women needing services for abortion or for management of abortion complications that cannot be provided on site

District hospital level

- All elements of abortion care mentioned for the primary-care level
- Provision of sterilization in addition to other contraceptive methods
- Abortion services for all circumstances and stages of pregnancy in which it is permitted by law
- Management of abortion complications
- Information and outreach programmes covering the full catchment area
- Training of all relevant cadres of health professionals (pre-service and in-service) in abortion service provision

Referral hospitals (secondary and tertiary)

- All elements of abortion care mentioned for the previous levels
- Management of all abortion complications, including those that cannot be managed at district level

2.2   ESSENTIAL EQUIPMENT, SUPPLIES, MEDICATIONS AND FACILITY CAPABILITIES

The following table (Table 3.2) gives a summary of what is needed for providing abortion services at different levels of the health care system. Most of the supplies, equipment and infrastructure needed for vacuum aspiration and medical methods of abortion are the same as those needed for gynaecological care and for clinical contraception. A detailed list of essential equipment and supplies for the provision of manual vacuum aspiration is included in Annex 3. Details about the drugs needed for the management of complications, such as oxytocin, IV fluids and antibiotics, can be found elsewhere (World Health Organization 2000).

These instruments and medications should be routinely included in the planning, budgeting, procurement, distribution and management systems. Criteria for determining what instruments to use are: quality, durability, system ability to ensure consistent availability and maintenance over time, and cost.

The introduction of vacuum aspiration can help health systems increase the availability of and accessibility to abortion since its ease of use makes it appropriate for facilities at the primary health care level. In addition, the costs are relatively low (Lean et al. 1976). Costing studies of manual vacuum aspiration have been carried out on its introduction for treating complications of unsafe abortion. These demonstrate substantial reduction in costs from the use of manual vacuum aspiration as well as improved quality of care (Anonymous 2000, Brambila et al. 1999, El Shafei et al. 1999). Programmatic and resource considerations may influence decisions about which method of vacuum aspiration to offer. In hospital settings and other sites that perform a high volume of abortions, the use of electric vacuum aspiration may be more efficient than manual vacuum aspiration. However, where electric vacuum aspiration is being used and where electrical power supply is unreliable, back-up availability of manual vacuum aspiration is essential. Vacuum aspiration has proven highly acceptable to providers in different settings (Bradley et al. 1991, Ekwempu 1990, Population Council 2000a, Population Council 2000b, University of North Carolina 2001).

Table 3.2 Instruments, medications and facility requirements for abortion

Method	Instruments and medication	Facility requirements
Vacuum aspiration	- Basic gynaecological and medical instruments and supplies (e.g., open speculum, ring or sponge forceps, antiseptic solution, gauze or swabs, gloves), tenaculum - Mechanical dilators (Pratt or Denniston), osmotic dilators, or misoprostol for cervical dilation - Needles and local anaesthetic for paracervical block - Analgesics - Suction: manual or electric vacuum aspirator and tubing - Cannulae: flexible or rigid, angled or straight; different sizes - Sieve and glass bowl for tissue inspection	- Instruments and medication - Private area for counselling - Clean treatment area offering privacy - Examination table with leg supports or stirrups - Bed - Stool for provider - Clean water - Strong lighting - Supplies for decontamination and cleaning and high-level disinfection of instruments - Disposable waste container - Adequate toilet facilities
Medical methods of abortion	Basic gynaecological and medical instruments and supplies (e.g. open speculum, gauze or swabs, menstrual pads, gloves) Depending on the protocol used: - Mifepristone + misoprostol or gemeprost - Analgesics - Glass bowl for tissue inspection	- Private area for counselling - Private area with chairs to wait for expulsion separate from women giving birth - Adequate toilet facilities - Capacity to provide or refer for vacuum aspiration
D&E	All items listed for vacuum aspiration and: - Larger dilators and large bore cannula - Special forceps (eg. Sopher or Bierer) for later procedures - Oxytocin	All those listed for vacuum aspiration

Safe Abortion: Technical and Policy Guidance for Health Systems

Instruments for manual vacuum aspiration are made for either single use or multiple use. Where instruments will be reused, it is essential to purchase those that can withstand multiple use and cleaning. Instruments for single use offer the advantage of ensuring sterility of equipment and thus of safety to the woman, as well as being convenient for the provider. The disadvantage is that supplies cost more and must be regularly available. They also need to be carefully disposed of to avoid health risks to providers and the community. Reusable equipment saves costs in terms of supplies, but rigorous cleaning and disinfection procedures must be followed (see Chapter 2, section 2.5.1).

2.2.1 Regulatory requirements for drugs and devices

Each country has specific regulatory requirements for the registration and importation of drugs. However, WHO's Model List of Essential Medicines, which has been adapted by many countries as a National Essential Drugs List, includes non-narcotic analgesics such as non-steroidal anti-inflammatory agents (e.g. ibuprofen), tranquillisers (e.g. diazepam) and local anaesthetics (lidocaine) (World Health Organization 2002b). Inclusion on the National Essential Drug List usually means that the drug is registered and available in the country. Where a drug is not registered, some countries will allow importation through the WHO Certification Scheme on the Quality of Pharmaceutical Products Moving in International Commerce (see Annex 1 for online information).

Some countries, but not all, also have registration requirements for medical devices. Programme managers should check whether product registration is required before importation of devices such as manual vacuum aspiration kits.

The commodities included in Table 3.2 that are specific to the provision of abortion services should be included in the national medical supplies logistics management programme and be available for those health facilities that require them.

2.3 REFERRAL MECHANISMS

It is extremely important for the provision of safe abortion services that a well-functioning referral system be in place. All health centre, clinic or hospital staff should be able to direct women to appropriate services if they are not available on site. Referral and transport arrangements among various levels of the health care system are necessary to ensure that (a) women who need services can obtain them in a timely manner, and (b) women who need care for complications of unsafe abortion receive treatment promptly. If women presenting with an unwanted pregnancy are not eligible for a legal abortion, it is essential that health care providers are able to offer support, information and/or advice to help them make plans for the continuation of the pregnancy and referral for prenatal care.

Key elements in a functioning referral and transport system include:

- standard procedures for determining when referral is necessary and how to make referrals, including arrangements for transport;

- standard procedures for facilities to accept and treat women who are referred and for reporting back to the referring centre;

- guidelines on handling patient information to ensure both safe and appropriate care, as well as confidentiality;

- guidelines for assessing clients' needs for referral to other types of services, such as STI or HIV services, social services or counselling, and judicial services for women who have suffered rape.

2.4 RESPECT FOR WOMEN'S INFORMED DECISION-MAKING, AUTONOMY, CONFIDENTIALITY AND PRIVACY, WITH ATTENTION TO THE SPECIAL NEEDS OF ADOLESCENTS

National norms, standards and regulations should support both women's ability to exercise their reproductive and other rights, and health care workers' fulfilment of their ethical obligations. Within the framework of national abortion laws, norms and standards should include protection for: informed and free decision-making, autonomy in decision-making, confidentiality and privacy (Cook and Dickens 2000). These standards are reinforced by international human rights standards contained in, amongst others, the International Covenant on Economic, Social and Cultural Rights, and the Convention on the Elimination of All Forms of Discrimination Against Women.

2.4.1 Informed and free decision-making

Women trying to resolve the problem of an unwanted pregnancy may often feel they are in a vulnerable position, especially vis-à-vis the health services. They need to be treated with respect and understanding. Health providers should therefore be supportive of the woman and give her information in a way that she can understand and recall, so that she can make a choice about having or not having an abortion to the extent permitted by law, free of inducement, coercion or discrimination.

Health providers should also be aware of situations in which a woman may be coerced into having an abortion against her will, based, for instance, on her health status such as being infected with HIV. In such cases, the provider should endeavour to ensure fully informed and free decision-making.

Health workers have a right to conscientious objection to providing abortion, but they have an ethical obligation to follow professional ethical codes, which usually require health professionals to refer women to skilled colleagues who are not, in principle, opposed to termination of pregnancy allowed by law. If no alternative provider is available, the health worker must provide abortion to save the woman's life or to prevent permanent damage to her health in accordance with national law.

When a hospital, clinic or health centre has been designated as a public facility offering services allowed by law, it cannot endanger women's lives or health by refusing services. It should provide abortion services on the grounds allowed by the law.

2.4.2 Autonomy in decision-making (third party authorization)

The fundamental ethical principle of respect for persons includes respecting their autonomy. Autonomy means that mentally competent adults do not require the consent (authorization) of any third party, such as a husband or partner, to access a health service. Therefore, health providers should not impose a requirement of spousal authorization unless required by enacted law and related regulations.

Respect for persons also includes the obligation to protect vulnerable people. Unmarried women, adolescents, those living in extreme poverty and those facing violence in the home, may be considered particularly vulnerable. Stigma and discrimination associated with physical and mental disabilities and health status such as HIV infection are widespread and may be used as a reason to coerce women into having an abortion. Health providers have an ethical obligation to ensure that such women receive necessary health services.

In regard to parental consent (authorization) for minors, nearly all Governments have ratified the Convention on the Rights of the Child (CRC). Article 5 of the Convention provides that "States parties shall respect the responsibilities, rights and duties of parents…to provide, in a manner consistent with the evolving capacities of the child, appropriate direction and guidance in the exercise by the child of rights recognised in the present Convention." In addition, however, Article 3, which contains one of four guiding general principles that govern the implementation of all articles of the Convention, states that, "In all actions concerning children [defined as every human being below the age of 18 years] whether undertaken by public or private social welfare institutions, courts of law, administrative authorities or legislative bodies, the best interest of the child shall be a primary consideration."

Special considerations for adolescents

Adolescents often lack knowledge about sexuality, contraception, how pregnancy occurs, what the signs of pregnancy are, and sexually transmitted infections. Young and unmarried adolescents in particular may not admit to having had sex and thus the possibility of pregnancy. They may have limited experience in talking to adults on such matters and in accessing and using health services to address their sexual health and reproductive health needs. Adolescents need a supportive environment in which they can express their needs, fears and embarrassment without being judged or "talked down" to.

Health care providers must overcome their possible discomfort with adolescent sexuality, particularly of unmarried adolescents, since it is a reality in most places. They also need knowledge and appropriate skills to handle adolescents which include special history-taking skills. For instance, they should be gentle and ask simple questions in plain language. They may need to repeat questions, and probe carefully and with consideration. They may have to suggest different responses to encourage adolescents to speak since adolescents often need time to reveal their problems. It is essential that service providers clearly guarantee confidentiality by ensuring the adolescent that they will not share the information about her visit to the health centre with anyone.

"Adolescent-friendly" health services may need to be developed to ensure that adolescents have access to needed services. Frequently this can be achieved by reorienting existing services to better meet the needs of adolescents. This might involve ensuring services are open at times and places where adolescents can reach them, and ensuring that fees are affordable. The existence of such services must be made known to adolescents and their families, and community support is often helpful for this.

(World Health Organization, 2002c)

2 Establishing national norms and standards *continued*

Health workers should encourage minors to consult parents or another trusted adult about their pregnancy. If the girl indicates that is not possible (e.g. a parent is abusive), service providers should not require parental consent, unless required by enacted law and related regulations. Health care providers need to be trained on how to inform, counsel and treat adolescents according to their evolving capacities to understand the treatment and care options being offered, and not according to some arbitrary age cut-off.

2.4.3 Confidentiality

Providers have a duty to protect patients' information against unauthorized disclosures, and to ensure that patients who do authorize release of their confidential information to others do so freely and on the basis of clear information.

The fear that confidentiality will not be maintained deters many women – particularly adolescents and unmarried women – from seeking health care services and may drive them to clandestine and dangerous providers or to self-induced abortion. Unless the woman explicitly approves a provider's consultation with her spouse or parent or anyone else not essential to ensure safe and appropriate care, such consultation constitutes a serious breach of confidentiality.

2.4.4 Privacy

To the maximum extent possible, health service managers should ensure that facilities provide privacy for conversations between women and providers, as well as for actual services. Privacy can be accomplished, at a minimum, by, for example, providing a single procedure per room at any one time, putting up curtains on windows and doorways, and providing a simple cloth or paper drapes for the woman for the procedure.

2.5 SPECIAL PROVISIONS FOR WOMEN WHO HAVE SUFFERED RAPE

Women who are pregnant as a result of rape are in need of particularly sensitive treatment, and all levels of the health system should be able to offer appropriate care and support.

Norms and standards for provision of abortion in such cases should be elaborated and training provided. Such standards should not impose unnecessary administrative or judicial procedures such as requiring women to press charges or to identify the rapist (Billings et al. 2002) (see also Chapter 4). The standards should ideally also be part of comprehensive norms and standards for the overall management of survivors of rape, covering physical and psychological care, emergency contraception, treatment for STIs or injuries, collecting forensic evidence, and counselling and follow-up care (World Health Organization and United Nations High Commissioner for Refugees 2002).

3 Ensuring provider skills and performance

3.1 PROVIDER SKILLS AND TRAINING

Making safe, legal abortion services accessible to all eligible women is likely to require involving midlevel health professionals because trained medical doctors are not sufficiently available in many parts of the world. In a number of countries midlevel providers such as midwives and other skilled health care workers who are not physicians have been trained to deliver quality postabortion care and abortion care (Billings et al. 1999, Dickson-Tetteh et al. 2000, Population Council 2000b, University of North Carolina 2001, Yumkella and Githiori 2000). A comparative study has shown no difference in complication rates between women who had first trimester abortions with manual vacuum aspiration performed by a physician assistant and those who had the procedure performed by a physician (Freedman et al. 1986).

Health workers already competent to provide basic abortion services can be trained to provide more complex care. For example, health workers who perform abortions for pregnancies up to nine weeks' duration can be taught to perform abortions for later stages of pregnancy. Providers who perform vacuum aspiration for treatment of incomplete abortion can learn to use the technique for safe abortion with modest additional training.

Skills training required for provision of safe abortion should be included into pre- and in-service curricula of health providers who are allowed to provide abortion services. Skills for the recognition and management of complications of abortion should be included in the curricula for all health care providers who treat women. All staff should also receive periodic updating in these skills.

Midlevel providers refers to a range of non-physician clinicians – midwives, nurse practitioners, clinical officers, physician assistants, and others – whose training and responsibilities differ among countries but who are trained to provide basic, clinical procedures related to reproductive health including bimanual pelvic examination to determine pregnancy and positioning of the uterus, uterine sounding, transcervical procedures, and who can be trained to provide an early abortion. [Definition proposed and agreed upon by participants at the Technical Consultation in September 2000.]

3 Ensuring provider skills and performance *continued*

3.1.1 Training programmes

Training programmes, both pre- and in-service, should be based on a competency approach including supervised practice sufficient to allow the health practitioner to demonstrate clinical competence. Programmes should use a variety of teaching and learning methodologies and should address both technical and clinical skills as well as attitudes and beliefs of the service provider. This may require a values clarification process which allows health providers to differentiate between their own values and the rights of the client to receive quality services. Programmes must be conducted in facilities that have sufficient patient flow to allow all trainees to have the requisite practice, including practice in managing complications.

Curricula may vary in content as well as length of training depending on the skills the health provider already has on entry into the training programme (see Table 3.3 for full list of essential content). All training must ensure that the health practitioner is competent to:

- Use a wide range of interpersonal communication skills to establish effective rapport and communication with all service users, respecting their human right to be treated with dignity and respect, and to confidentiality;

- Effectively transmit and discuss sensitive information regarding sexual behaviour and pregnancy;

- Enable clients to make informed decisions;

- Conduct a safe and accurate bimanual pelvic examination to diagnose pregnancy, as well as size and position of the uterus and to reach an appropriate decision to carry out an abortion or refer to a higher level of service;

- Recognise or suspect ectopic pregnancy;

- Accurately recognize the signs and symptoms of RTIs and STIs;

- Recognise signs of physical abuse;

- Administer drugs correctly;

- Accurately carry out the abortion procedure(s) for which they are being trained;

- Take effective action in case of complications before, during or after the procedure;

- Make effective referrals to other appropriate services;

- Provide contraceptive information and services;

- Clean and ensure safety of all equipment used for the procedure;

- Make accurate records.

Table 3.3 lists recommended training content for all health professionals. Details of training curricula and related resource materials are included in Annex 1.

Table 3.3 **Essential content for curricula on abortion services**

Background for abortion service delivery

- Legal, regulatory and policy provisions
- Health effects of unsafe abortion

- Ethical responsibility to provide abortion
- National norms and standards for abortion care

Counselling and provider-patient interaction

- Clarification of providers' attitudes and beliefs with regard to abortion
- Privacy and confidentiality
- Interpersonal communication and counselling skills
- Information on abortion and contraception

- Issues and risks associated with HIV and other STIs
- Groups needing special care, such as adolescents, refugees, women with HIV or STI infection
- Recognition of signs that the woman has been subjected to violence, and guidance in helping her obtain additional counselling and services

Clinical skills

- Anatomy and physiology relevant to pregnancy and abortion
- Pre-procedure assessment: history, examinations, pregnancy dating, etc.
- STI screening
- Abortion techniques
- Infection prevention

- Pain management
- Recognition and management of, and/or referral for, complications of abortion
- Management and care following the procedure, including contraceptive information and services
- Criteria for referral and how to refer cases beyond the provider's competence

Administrative/managerial issues and quality assurance

- Record-keeping and reporting
- Conditions for maintaining privacy and confidentiality
- Logistics, equipment and inventory management

- Monitoring and evaluation
- Mechanisms for effective referral and transport to qualified facilities
- Standards for supervision

3 Ensuring provider skills and performance *continued*

3.2 SUPERVISION

The service system must enable supervisors to ensure that service delivery meets norms and standards, satisfies clients' needs and respects their rights. Supervisors' duties include:

- creating a respectful environment by demonstrating supportive attitudes and behaviour towards providers and clients;

- assigning jobs and tasks to health workers with appropriate skills and monitoring their work to ensure both technical quality and compassionate care;

- ensuring providers' access to the necessary equipment, commodities, and spaces to provide counselling and services assuring privacy and confidentiality;

- monitoring the need for, and ensuring, in-service training of staff;

- monitoring and ensuring access to services without discrimination on the basis of, for instance, age or marital status, or that no unauthorized charges are made; and

- ensuring fully informed and free consent about abortion and post-abortion contraception.

An important tool for supervision can be a checklist of items that supervisors are to monitor regularly (see Table 3.4). Such a checklist needs to be developed locally to reflect particular circumstances, and administered so as to maintain quality of care.

Table 3.4 **Categories for inclusion in supervisor checklist**

- Equipment (availability, amount, condition, cleaning, sterilization, storage)
- Supplies (adequate, not outdated, stored appropriately)
- Observation of counselling given
- Observation of clinical services
- Provisions for privacy
- Cleanliness of the facility
- Accuracy and completeness of records
- Review of statistical records and patient files for completeness
- Analysis of basic service statistics

3.3 CERTIFICATION AND LICENSING OF HEALTH PROFESSIONALS AND FACILITIES

Where certification of abortion providers is required, its sole purpose should be to ensure that providers meet essential criteria for the safe provision of care, as with other medical procedures. Certification and licensing requirements should not be used to exclude categories of health professionals. As mentioned in section 3.1 above, many different categories of health providers can be trained to provide safe abortion.

In those countries in which facilities offering abortion are licensed, the licensing requirements must meet the nationally agreed criteria. Facility licensing is to ensure client safety and comprehensiveness of care. However, such licensing requirements should not impose excessive requirements for sophisticated equipment, infrastructure or staff that are not essential to provision of safe services and would unnecessarily restrict access.

4 Monitoring and evaluation of services

As with all health services, abortion services should be subject to quality monitoring and evaluation. The regular and accurate collection of service statistics and regular monitoring and evaluation at the facility level are a key to maintaining and improving the quality of services delivered. They can also help in assessing whether abortion services are actually available to those women eligible by law. Over time, if baseline information has been collected, including data on mortality and morbidity from unsafe abortion, and if basic service statistics are routinely and accurately kept, programmes will be able to evaluate the extent to which full access to legal services reduces maternal mortality and morbidity. These statistics and other information gathered through monitoring and evaluation should be shared and discussed with stakeholders and used to make decisions about improvements to services.

4.1 MONITORING

Monitoring oversees the processes of implementing services, including changes over time. Routine monitoring can assist managers and supervisors to identify and manage or avoid problems before they become serious or overwhelming. Good monitoring includes listening to providers who can have important recommendations to improve quality of care. Well designed monitoring enables facility managers and staff supervisors to give feedback to staff on problems and to engage staff in a participatory process to implement solutions. At the facility level, processes and mechanisms for monitoring services include case reviews, logbook review, observation, checklists, facility surveys and maternal death audits, all of which can be used to improve quality of care (see Annex 1 for further reading).

4 Monitoring and evaluation of services *continued*

As far as feasible, service-delivery facilities should integrate data on abortion services into regular record systems (e.g. forms, logbooks, supply stock records, checklists, clinical client records, daily activity registers) rather than create separate ones. Basic service statistics include, at a minimum, a record of abortions provided, women seen but not provided with services, women referred to higher levels of care, treatment of complications of abortion and contraceptive methods accepted. The amount and types of service statistics required to be recorded should be suited to the ability and workloads of staff. It is more valuable to have a narrow range of accurate data with a good feedback mechanism than to impose reporting requirements that staff are unable or unwilling to meet.

Selected facility-level data should be sent routinely to higher levels to enable monitoring across facilities and geographic areas, and should be used at the national level for informing policy and planning.

It can also be very useful to monitor the costs to the health facility of providing legal abortion and of treating complications of unsafe abortion.

Routine monitoring should include:

- Analysis of patterns or problems in services using service statistics (e.g. numbers of women seen but not provided with services, numbers of complications, numbers of contraceptive methods provided by type)

- Proportion of women seeking repeat abortions

- Observation of counselling and clinical services to assess quality of interaction with the woman throughout the process, to correct any shortfalls in adherence to technical standards, or other practices that jeopardise quality of care (e.g. judgmental attitudes, imposition of "informal charges")

- Functioning of logistics system to ensure regular supply of equipment and consumables

- Regular aggregation of data from facility level upwards

- Assessment of progress to remedy problems identified in routine monitoring.

Table 3.5 **Suggested data sources and indicators for monitoring and evaluating abortion services**

Routine service statistics

- Numbers of abortions provided, by completed week of pregnancy and by type of procedure
- Time between first consultation and abortion
- Number of women referred elsewhere, by reason
- Number of women seen but not provided with services, by reason
- Number of women treated for complications, by type of abortion procedure
- Contraceptives provided, by type
- Referrals for contraception

Periodic evaluation

- Percentage of service delivery points offering abortion care, and their distribution by geographic area and level of the health care system, and patterns of utilization
- Number of providers performing abortion and their distribution by geographic area and level of the health system
- Number of health workers trained, by type; assessment of quality of training
- Assessment of quality of care provided
- Costs of abortion services and of treating the complications of abortion, by type of procedure and type of provider, and any fees charged
- Periodic special studies (client satisfaction, proximity of women to facilities, costs, impact, etc.)
- Number of staff needing in-service training and numbers trained

Patient information (kept in patient file)

- Age, parity, marital status
- Reason(s) for referral
- Reason(s) for refusal
- Follow-up care given
- Contraceptive method chosen
- Fee charged, if any

4.2 EVALUATION

Evaluation assesses the relevance, effectiveness, efficiency, sustainability and impact of services using service statistics from monitoring, as well as special investigations to assess the extent to which programme goals are being accomplished. For example, has quality improved? Are all eligible women gaining access? Are quantitative and qualitative training objectives being met? Has the number of service delivery points increased? Evaluations can be conducted at health centre level, regional or sub-regional and national levels and should be designed early in programme development to include both a baseline assessment and scheduled evaluation points.

Periodic, client-based evaluations to assess women's experiences, complications, quality of care received, and access to services will provide important information for improving clinic and outreach services. This can be done with questionnaires, observation guides, and exit interviews. Similar evaluations should also be carried out with providers, to assess their attitudes, knowledge, practices, needs and ideas for improving services.

Impact evaluations can measure the extent to which improved access to and quality of services for eligible women help to meet health goals. For example, periodic special studies of a sample of facilities and catchment areas can assess increases in the use of legal services. Special studies could also examine changes in hospital admissions for complications of unsafe abortion before and after improvements are made. Like other evaluations, assessment of impact requires a strong baseline assessment and clear specification of programme objectives and indicators.

In most instances, it is more important to define a few clearly measurable indicators than to attempt to collect a comprehensive list of data, especially where health system research capacity is limited. Where capacity is strong, a more comprehensive approach may be desirable. Evaluations should include not only quantifiable indicators but also qualitative assessments. The latter can include interviews with providers, women, men and community leaders to determine their knowledge of services and eligibility, their perceived need for services, and their views about existing services.

5 Financing

Health service budgets should include costs of:

- Instruments, supplies and medications needed to begin offering abortion or to improve existing services throughout the system (see Chapter 2)

- Staff time (whether part time or full time)

- Training programmes

- One-time (usually modest) capital costs such as renovating a treatment space.

Because safe abortion services do not require additional skills or equipment from those that should already be available for obstetrical and gynaecological care, the additional costs of making such services available to eligible women are likely to be modest given the gains for women's health. Most national health budgets should be able to cover these costs.

If user fees, medical insurance or other cost-recovery measures are applied to abortion care, they must be designed so as not to impede women's access to services.

5.1   COST TO THE FACILITY OR HEALTH SYSTEM

Costs include infrequent, modest capital investments as well as recurrent costs. Examples of infrequent capital costs are purchases of items such as a suction machine, an examination table, a sterilizer or an autoclave; construction or renovation of consultation and treatment rooms. Recurrent costs include those associated with purchasing instruments and supplies that will need to be restocked regularly, such as cannulae, manual vacuum aspirators, drugs, gauze, antiseptic solutions and cold sterilants used for instrument processing; other recurrent costs include ongoing training, staffing and facility operations. As mentioned earlier, most of these items are likely to be available already in facilities serving pregnant women.

Decisions about which abortion methods to offer and how to organize services directly influence the cost of providing services and their affordability.
Two organizational issues are of particular importance. First, as mentioned earlier, switching from D&C to vacuum aspiration for uterine evacuation is not only safer for the woman but has been shown to reduce health system costs substantially (Jowett 2000). Vacuum aspiration can be performed in a simple outpatient treatment room by a trained midlevel health worker, whereas D&C requires an operating theatre and a physician. Vacuum aspiration usually requires less medication for pain than D&C because it is less painful (Grimes et al. 1977) and women can leave the health care facility sooner. Second, as the health system effectively informs women to come early in pregnancy, the use of lower-cost, early procedures goes up and that of the costlier later procedures goes down. These and other changes in patient management not only reduce costs but also improve quality of care.

5.2   MAKING SERVICES AFFORDABLE FOR WOMEN

Facilities often set fees for services so high as to make them unaffordable for many women. Some publicly financed programmes that provide other types of health care free to poor women do not cover abortion or pay only for certain types of procedures. In addition, women may be expected to pay substantial "informal charges" (charges made by providers on top of the official health system charges) which, combined with travel expenses and opportunity costs such as time lost from paid employment, pose a barrier many women cannot cross. Practices such as these are likely to cost the health system more money in the long run by increasing the number of women who attempt to induce abortion themselves or go to unsafe providers, and end up hospitalized with serious complications.

5   Financing *continued*

Where fees are charged for abortion, such fees should be matched to women's ability to pay and should not limit access for women who cannot pay, including low-income women and adolescents. Furthermore, all facilities should have procedures in place to ensure that "informal" charges are not imposed by staff. Other steps that can be taken to make abortion services more affordable for women include subsidizing abortion services for poor women with revenue from other services or from higher-income women; reducing fee differentials for abortions performed at different durations of pregnancy and among different methods, so that women can access services that best suit their needs without regard to cost; and providing information about the availability of abortion services and any associated fees, so that women can make decisions based on accurate knowledge of cost. Abortion should never be denied or delayed because of a woman's inability to pay.

References

Anonymous. (2000) Improving quality and reducing costs in post-abortion care in Peru. *Reproductive Health Matters* 8:189.

Billings DL, Ankrah V, Baird TL, Taylor JE, Ababio KP and Ntow S. (1999) Midwives and comprehensive postabortion care in Ghana. In Huntington D and Piet-Pelon NJ (eds). Postabortion care: lessons from operations research. New York, Population Council, pp 141-158.

Billings DL, Moreno C, Ramos C, González de León D, Ramirez R, Martinez LV and Díaz MR. (2002) Constructing access to legal abortion services in Mexico City. *Reproductive Health Matters* 10(19):87-95.

Bradley J, Sikazwe N and Healy J. (1991) Improving abortion care in Zambia. *Studies in Family Planning* 22:391-394.

Brambila C, Langer A, Garcia-Barrios C and Heimburger A. (1999) Estimating costs of postabortion services at Dr Aurelio Valdivieso General Hospital, Oaxaca, Mexico. In Huntington D and Piet-Pelon NJ (eds). *Postabortion care: lessons from operations research.* New York, Population Council, pp 108-124.

Cook R and Dickens B. (2000) *Considerations for formulating reproductive health laws.* Second edition. Geneva, World Health Organization. (WHO/RHR/00.1)

Coyaji K. (2000) Early medical abortion in India: three studies and their implications for abortion services. *Journal of American Medical Women's Association* 55(Suppl):191-194.

Dickson-Tetteh K, Mavuya LM, Gabriel M, Rees H, Billings DL and King TDN. (2000) *Abortion care services provided by registered midwives in South Africa: a report on the midwifery training program.* Johannesburg, Reproductive Health Research Unit and Ipas.

Ekwempu CC. (1990) Uterine aspiration using the Karman cannula and syringe. *Tropical Journal of Obstetrics and Gynaecology* 8:37-38.

El Shafei M, Hassan EO, Mashalli A, Shalan H and El Lakkany N. (1999) Improving reproductive health service by using manual vacuum aspiration in the management of incomplete abortion. *Egyptian Society of Obstetrics and Gynecology* 25:711-722.

Freedman MA, Jillson D, Coffin RR and Novick LF. (1986) Comparison of complication rates in first trimester abortions performed by physician assistants and physicians. *American Journal of Public Health* 76:550-554.

Greenslade FC, Benson J, Winkler J, Henderson V, Wolf M and Leonard A. (1993) Summary of clinical and programmatic experience with manual vacuum aspiration. *IPAS Advances in Abortion Care* 3(2):1-4.

Grimes D, Schulz KF, Cates W and Tyler CW. (1977) The Joint Program for the Study of Abortion/ CDC: a preliminary report. In Hern W and Andrikopolous B (eds). *Abortion in the seventies.* New York, National Abortion Federation, pp. 41-46.

Jowett M. (2000) Safe motherhood interventions in low-income countries: an economic justification and evidence of cost effectiveness. *Health Policy* 53:201-228.

King TD, Abernathy M, Hord C, Nicholson LA, Benson J and Johnson BR. (1998) *A guide to assessing resource use in the provision of postabortion care.* Carrboro, Ipas.

Lawson HW, Frye A, Atrash HK, Smith JC, Shulman HB and Ramick M. (1994) Abortion mortality, United States: 1972 through 1987. *American Journal of Obstetrics and Gynecology* 171:1365-1372.

Lean TH, Vengadasalam D, Pachauri S and Miller ET. (1976) A comparison of D&C and vacuum aspiration for performing first trimester abortion. *International Journal of Gynecology and Obstetrics* 14:481-486.

Mundigo AI and Indriso C (eds). (1999) *Abortion in the developing world.* New Delhi, Visitaar Publications for the World Health Organization.

Population Council. (2000a) *Burkina Faso: postabortion care. Upgrading postabortion care benefits patients and providers.* Washington DC, Population Council, Frontiers in Reproductive Health.

Population Council. (2000b) *Senegal: postabortion care. Train more providers in postabortion care.* Washington DC, Population Council, Frontiers in Reproductive Health.

RCOG - Royal College of Obstetricians and Gynaecologists. (2000) *The care of women requesting induced abortion.* Evidence-based guideline No.7. London, RCOG Press.

University of North Carolina. (2001) *PRIME postabortion care.* Chapel Hill, University of North Carolina, Program for International Training in Health (INTRAH).

Veira Villela W and de Oliveira Araujo MJ. (2000) Making legal abortion available in Brazil: partnerships in practice. *Reproductive Health Matters* 8(16):77-82.

World Health Organization. (1999) *Abortion in Viet Nam: an assessment of policy, programme and research issues.* Geneva, World Health Organization. (WHO/RHR/HRP/IRR/99.2)

World Health Organization. (2000) *Managing the complications of pregnancy and childbirth: a guide for midwives and doctors.* Geneva, World Health Organization. (WHO/RHR/00.7)

World Health Organization. (2002a) *Making decisions about contraceptive introduction. A guide for conducting assessments to broaden contraceptive choice and improve quality of care.* Geneva, World Health Organization. (WHO/RHR/02.11)

World Health Organization. (2002b) Essential medicines: WHO model list (12th Edition). Geneva, World Health Organization. Available on-line at: *http://www.who.int/medicines/organization/par/edl/expertcomm.shtml*

World Health Organization. (2002c) *Global consultation on adolescent friendly health services. A consensus statement.* Geneva, World Health Organization. (WHO/FCH/02.18)

World Health Organization and United Nations High Commissioner for Refugees. (2002) *Clinical management of survivors of rape. A guide to the development of protocols for use in refugee and internally displaced person situations.* Geneva, World Health Organization and United Nations High Commissioner for Refugees. (WHO/RHR/02.08)

Yumkella F and Githiori F. (2000) *Expanding opportunities for postabortion care at the community level through private nurse-midwives in Kenya.* Chapel Hill, University of North Carolina, Program for International Training in Health (INTRAH).

Chapter **4** Legal and policy considerations

Chapter 4 Summary

- Unsafe abortion is one of the main causes of maternal mortality and morbidity even though it is legal for a variety of circumstances in almost all countries. This is because safe abortion services are frequently not available even when it would be legal to provide them. The ICPD + 5 review and appraisal process agreed that, in circumstances where abortion is not against the law, "health systems should train and equip health service providers and take other measures to ensure that such abortion is safe and accessible". Understanding the circumstances under which abortion is not against the law, and the related policy considerations, is crucial for implementing this mandate.

- In almost all countries abortion is allowed at least when there is a threat to the woman's life. The majority of national laws also allow abortion when pregnancy poses a threat to the woman's physical or mental health; many allow it when pregnancy is the result of rape or incest or when there is fetal impairment. Many laws also allow abortion for socioeconomic reasons, and on request by the woman.

- An enabling policy environment is needed to ensure that every woman legally eligible has ready access to good-quality abortion services. Policies should be geared to achieving positive health outcomes for women, to providing good-quality family planning information and services, and to meeting the particular needs of groups such as poor women, adolescents, rape survivors and HIV-infected women.

- Policies and programmes should remove barriers to timely provision of services. Such barriers include lack of public knowledge of the law and where to obtain legal abortion services; third-party authorization or notification clauses; hindering and unnecessary conditions or procedures such as waiting periods or lack of privacy; and excessive restrictions on the kinds of health professionals or institutions licensed to provide abortion. Table 4.2 on pages 91-94 lists some common barriers and suggests actions to correct them.

1 Women's health and international agreements

The great majority of the deaths from unsafe abortion occur in developing countries where abortion is severely restricted by law (Alan Guttmacher Institute 1999). In developing regions (excluding China), 330 deaths occur per 100,000 abortions, a mortality rate that is hundreds of times higher than the rate in developed countries. The rate is highest – an estimated 680 deaths per 100,000 procedures – in Africa (Alan Guttmacher Institute 1999, World Health Organization 1998).

Most Governments have ratified legally-binding international treaties and conventions that protect human rights, including the right to the highest attainable standard of health, the right to non-discrimination, the right to life, liberty and security of the person, the right to be free from inhuman and degrading treatment, and the right to education and information.

In consideration of these human rights, Governments agreed in the ICPD+5 review and appraisal process that "…in circumstances where abortion is not against the law, health systems should train and equip health-service providers and should take other measures to ensure that such abortion is safe and accessible. Additional measures should be taken to safeguard women's health." (United Nations 1999, paragraph 63.iii). A clear understanding of laws on abortion as well as related policy considerations is required to ensure that all women eligible under the law have access to safe services. Further, the majority of the world's Governments at the 1995 Fourth World Conference on Women agreed they should "…consider reviewing laws containing punitive measures against women who have undergone illegal abortions." (United Nations 1996, paragraph 106).

2 Laws and their implementation

When a pregnancy threatens the woman's life, almost all countries permit abortion to save the woman's life, as indicated in Chapter 1, Figure 1.1 (United Nations Population Division 1999). Nearly two-thirds of countries allow abortion when there is serious risk to the woman's physical or mental health. In more than 40 per cent of countries, additional grounds for permitting abortion are rape or incest; and a similar percentage allow for abortion in cases of fetal impairment.

Many women seek abortion because they cannot afford to look after the child. In addition, there are many women – and this applies particularly to young, single women – for whom continuing a pregnancy would be socially difficult or impossible. In recognition of these problems, one-third of countries allow abortion on economic and/or social grounds. And some twenty-seven per cent of countries allow abortion on request, in recognition that all women seeking abortion face one or more of these problems.

2 Laws and their implementation *continued*

Abortion laws began to be liberalized in the first part of the twentieth century when the extent of the public health problem of unsafe abortion started to be recognized. Prosecutions for carrying out abortions began to disappear in the 1930s in some countries. In England, one medical practitioner deliberately provoked a court case against him in order to argue publicly in favour of decriminalization of abortion for public health reasons. Abortion laws began to be liberalized across Europe and in Canada, Cuba, India, the USA, Zambia and in several other countries in the 1960s and 1970s. Many other countries in all regions of the world have continued to reduce restrictions on and prosecutions for abortion, particularly since the mid-1980s (Berer 2000, Rahman et al. 1998).

The formulation of laws relating to abortion varies widely across countries, reflecting their diverse historical, political and religious roots (United Nations 2001a, 2001b, 2002). Provisions regarding abortion may be found in the criminal code, in civil law, or in both. In some countries, public health codes or medical ethics codes may contain special provisions that clarify how to interpret an abortion law but in many countries, no formalised interpretation or enabling regulation exists. In other countries, abortion may not be governed by an enacted law, but by a court interpretation. In a few countries, the existence of multiple texts may make it difficult at times to determine the exact meaning of the law and policy concerning abortion due to multiple or sometimes conflicting provisions. The elaboration and implementation of laws, policies and regulations reflect interpretation and involvement by various actors including courts, parliamentarians, policy-makers and health care providers, at various times. All of these factors affect both the availability of, and women's access to, safe, legal abortion services.

Research from a variety of countries indicates that women eligible under the law often are unable to obtain services (Gupte et al. 1997, Iyengar and Iyengar 2002, Koster-Oyekan 1998, Mundigo and Indriso 1999). The reasons include lack of training for providers, provider unwillingness, Government restrictions on types of facilities and providers who can carry out abortion or failure to provide them with the necessary authorization. They can also include a lack of resources for, and commitment to, delivering good-quality services at the primary care level (Berer 2000). In addition, many people – both health service providers as well as women – simply do not know what the law allows. For instance, in a region of one country where abortion is permitted up to 20 weeks of pregnancy, more than 75 per cent of married women and men were not aware that abortion was legal (Iyengar and Iyengar 2002). In countries with restrictive laws, health providers' cautious attitudes combined with often elaborate procedural requirements, are likely to make the approval process complicated and intimidating, particularly for women living in rural areas, young women and those who are illiterate (Alan Guttmacher Institute 1999).

There is thus considerable scope in most countries to:

- review and promote wider understanding of the relevant laws and policies;

- design and implement comprehensive policies to ensure access to services to the extent the law provides for;

- identify and remove unnecessary regulatory and administrative barriers to services.

3   Understanding legal grounds for abortion

It is essential for health professionals, and others such as police or court officers as well as the public, to have accurate information and to understand clearly what is allowed under the law in their country. While legal interpretations will always be specific to each country, some general remarks can be made regarding the circumstances under which abortion is most frequently allowed, as follows (United Nations 2001a, 2001b, 2002).

3.1   WHEN THERE IS A THREAT TO THE WOMAN'S LIFE

Almost all countries allow abortion to be performed to save the life of the pregnant woman. Some countries provide detailed lists of what they consider life-threatening situations. These lists are generally meant to provide illustrations of situations that are considered life-threatening, but they are not meant to preclude the doctor's clinical judgement of what is life-threatening for a particular woman. Such lists, however, may be interpreted restrictively, or be considered exhaustive, when in fact they are not. For example, if a list of physical dangers to life is considered exhaustive, that would exclude mental health conditions that are life-threatening.

All health personnel should know the high risks of maternal mortality and morbidity from unsafe abortion and they should be able to counsel women about legally allowed options. In some cases, physicians argue that it is necessary to provide a safe abortion because if they did not, the woman would risk her life by going to an unqualified practitioner (Oye-Adeniran et al. 2002).

Even where protecting a woman's life is the only allowable reason for abortion, it is essential that providers are trained, that services are available and known, and that treatment for complications of unsafe abortion is widely available along with family planning services.

3 Understanding legal grounds for abortion *continued*

3.2 WHEN THERE IS A THREAT TO THE WOMAN'S PHYSICAL OR MENTAL HEALTH

While "physical health" and "mental health" are sometimes separated as grounds for performing abortion, in many countries the law does not specify the aspects of health that are concerned but merely states that abortion is permitted to avert risk of injury to the pregnant woman's health. In such cases, the WHO definition of health – "a state of complete physical, mental and social well-being and not merely the absence of disease or infirmity" – has sometimes been applied (World Health Organization 2001).

When "mental health" is specifically mentioned in the law, some countries have interpreted "mental health" to include psychological distress caused by, for example, rape or incest, or by diagnosis of fetal impairment. In other circumstances, countries have also included in the interpretation of a threat to women's mental health, distress caused by detrimental socioeconomic circumstances.

3.3 WHEN PREGNANCY IS THE RESULT OF RAPE OR INCEST

In many countries, such cases are interpreted as falling within the mental health grounds for abortion. Some countries accept as evidence the woman's report. Others require forensic evidence of sexual penetration, or require evidence that intercourse was involuntary or

exploitative. For example, they may require that rape be established to the satisfaction of a judge who might require testimony from witnesses to a violation; or they may require that a police officer be convinced that the woman was violated before she obtains permission for the procedure to be undertaken.

These requirements, designed to screen out fabricated cases, often discourage women with legitimate grievances from seeking early, safe services. Delays due to judicial or police requirements can lead women to resort to clandestine, unsafe services or such delays can be so long drawn-out that the woman is ultimately denied abortion because her pregnancy is too advanced.

In such circumstances, judicial or administrative requirements should be minimized or removed, and clear protocols established for both police and health workers to facilitate prompt referral and access to appropriate care for women (Billings et al 2002, Veira Villela and de Oliveira Araujo 2000).

3.4 WHEN THERE IS FETAL IMPAIRMENT

This reason is increasingly permitted by countries with otherwise restrictive abortion laws because it is now possible to diagnose such conditions, many of which are considered to be incompatible with life, or independent life of the affected child. In some other countries, no specific reference is made in the law to fetal impairment; rather, mental health grounds are interpreted to include distress caused by diagnosis of fetal impairment.

3.5 FOR ECONOMIC AND SOCIAL REASONS

Most countries where abortion is permitted on economic and social grounds interpret the law to include the pregnant woman's social and economic environment, whether actual or foreseeable. Some assess whether the woman is in a state of distress as a result of her situation. Some laws include the extension of risk to cover any existing children of her family, that might be caused by an additional child.

3.6 ON REQUEST

A woman is allowed by law to obtain an abortion without giving a reason. Allowing abortion on request has emerged as countries have recognised that women seek abortions on one, and often more than one of the above grounds, and they accept all of these as legitimate.

3.7 LIMITS ON LENGTH OF PREGNANCY

Saving a woman's life might be necessary at any point during the pregnancy. Performing an abortion on grounds of fetal impairment is also likely to be in the second trimester since most such diagnoses can only be made after 12 weeks. Laws and policies that allow abortion for economic and social reasons, or on request, generally stipulate limits on the length of pregnancy. This is often 12 weeks since LMP. Some countries set the limit at 18, 22 or 24 weeks since LMP, while others do not specify length of pregnancy. Laws that include gestational limits usually permit abortion later in pregnancy in some circumstances or with additional requirements such as approval by two physicians rather than one (Alan Guttmacher Institute 1999, Rahman et al. 1998).

3.8 OTHER LIMITS

Abortion laws and policies sometimes unnecessarily restrict the kinds of facilities and practitioners allowed to perform abortion. They may also require authorization from other family members. These kinds of requirements, usually created to protect women's health, may have the opposite effect by creating insurmountable obstacles to access (Iyengar and Iyengar 2002, Koster-Oyekan 1998).

A law can also specify when abortion is illegal, rather than spelling out when it is legal. For instance, one such law specifies that abortion is illegal if done without the woman's consent; or done without accepted professional standards; or performed in an inadequate facility; or done for profit (Alvarez-Lajonchere 1989).

4 Creating an enabling policy environment

Policies take various forms and may include statutory regulations, regulations issued by the Ministry of Health, professional guidelines and training guidelines, among others. The central elements of a policy required to ensure access to safe abortion services

4   Creating an enabling policy environment *continued*

to the extent allowed by law are outlined below. While a comprehensive policy may not be immediately achievable, implementation of the ICPD (United Nations 1995) and ICPD+5 (United Nations 1999) agreements that legal abortion should be safe, ultimately requires action on all the elements listed in sections 4.1-4.7. Existing policies should be examined to ascertain where there are gaps and where improvements are needed.

4.1   GOALS

Policies should take account of prevailing national health service conditions and should aim to:

- minimize the rate of unwanted pregnancy and thus the recourse to abortion by providing good-quality family planning information and services, including emergency contraception;

- ensure that every woman legally eligible has ready access to safe abortion services;

- meet the particular needs of groups, such as poor women, adolescents, refugees and displaced women, HIV-infected women and survivors of rape, who may need special outreach and support.

In order to reach these goals, policies should address the following issues.

4.2   CONSTELLATION OF SERVICES

At a minimum, abortion services should always provide medically accurate information about abortion, and offer non-directive counselling and contraceptive information and services, as well as clinical abortion services (see Chapters 2 and 3 for details). Offering contraceptive information, services and referrals with abortion services, and with treatment for complications of unsafe abortion, helps prevent future unwanted pregnancy and reduce the need for abortion.

4.3   METHODS OF ABORTION

It is preferable to provide a choice of methods suited to health system capability as described in detail in Chapter 2. Even the most highly resource-constrained health systems should be able to provide manual vacuum aspiration safely for early abortion at all appropriate levels of the health care system and to refer women to higher levels of care when needed. Manual vacuum aspiration services should also be widely available to treat women who have complications of unsafe and incomplete abortion.

4.4   RANGE OF PROVIDERS

Laws usually require that abortions be undertaken by licensed medical practitioners. However, laws and policies governing medical procedures nearly always allow others, such as midlevel health care providers (e.g. midwives and nurses), to provide various medical services under supervision of a medical practitioner where necessary. Midlevel health workers can be trained to provide safe, early abortion. Training and equipping midlevel workers can help ensure appropriate service availability and accessibility without compromising safety, especially where doctors are few or not readily accessible (see Chapter 3).

4.5   SERVICE FEES

If official and "informal" fees for legal, safe abortion are high, they will increase the risk of recourse to unsafe abortion especially by poor women and others, such as adolescents, who do not have access to cash. Where fees for services and other charges are necessary, these should be kept as low and affordable as possible, and subsidies should be provided for those unable to pay. For public health services, the costs will likely be more than offset by the savings achieved by reducing unsafe abortion and the burden that complications of unsafe abortion impose on health systems.

4.6   HEALTH SYSTEM REQUIREMENTS/QUALITY OF CARE

Chapter 3 discusses curricula and standards, clinical and refresher training, logistics systems, management information systems, technical support services and supervision mechanisms, and health budget provisions. All these should be elaborated in an enabling policy.

It is essential that all health system personnel be given the necessary information required to inform women where and how to obtain legal services.

4.7   PUBLIC INFORMATION

Broad health education programmes should include basic information on how pregnancy occurs, the early signs of pregnancy, contraception and where and how to obtain legal abortion services (Table 4.1).

While many countries may require time to develop comprehensive policies, all countries can immediately take at least incremental steps to expand access to safe abortion services to the extent allowed by the law and to improve the quality of existing services as indicated below.

Table 4.1 **Core information for public education**

- Women have the *right to decide freely and responsibly* if and when to have children without coercion, discrimination or violence
- Basic *reproductive physiology*, including how pregnancy happens, its signs and symptoms
- How to *prevent unwanted pregnancy*, including where and how to obtain contraceptive methods
- *Circumstances* under which abortion is permitted
- The importance of seeking legal abortion services *as early as possible* when termination of pregnancy has been decided upon
- *Where and when* safe abortion is available, and its cost
- How to *recognize complications* of miscarriage and unsafe abortion; when and where to obtain treatment
- The importance of *seeking treatment immediately*.

5 Removing administrative and regulatory barriers

Often, certain regulations and guidance relating to the law may create barriers to accessing legal services. These barriers are not actually specified or required in the law itself. Some barriers evolve simply as a matter of practice and are mistakenly assumed to be legally required. All of these barriers are within the purview of Ministries of Health or professional associations to review and remove in order to ensure access to the extent allowed by the law. Ministries of Health can clarify legal requirements, inform personnel and end "common practices" that constrain access to services allowed by law. Table 4.2 provides examples of administrative, regulatory and other barriers that can be eliminated or modified to improve access to abortion services for eligible women.

Depending on the national context, the barriers listed in Table 4.2 may be imposed by regulatory requirements, or simply by administrative procedures. Some of the barriers listed in the left-hand column may have been requirements based on what is now outdated practice. For instance, the use of D&C may have generated restrictions on the types of personnel or institutions allowed to perform abortion that are not necessary when vacuum aspiration is introduced. Other barriers, such as requiring spousal authorization, authorized fees or waiting periods, are often administrative procedures imposed by providers. In such instances they may not be part of official policy nor required by law, nor are they necessary.

The gains for public health from removing the barriers are likely to be considerable. The middle column of Figure 4.2 describes illustrative actions to overcome the barriers. Often these are relatively straightforward, but in some cases, such as supporting public education, careful planning and investment of time and resources will be needed. The tasks implied by the "action" column are elaborated in various parts of this monograph. The third column – "rationale" – outlines the reasons for taking action, also dealt with in more detail throughout this guidance document.

Table 4.2 **Administrative and regulatory barriers to obtaining safe, legal abortion, and measures to eliminate these barriers**

Barriers	Possible actions	Rationale
Women and health professionals do not know the law or where to obtain legal abortion services.	Have governmental and other lawyers research and explain their understanding of the law. Support public education programmes. Include information about the law in training and updates for health professionals.	Lack of information is a major reason for women's recourse to unsafe abortion. Lack of knowledge about legal grounds for abortion causes providers to limit access.
Authorizations from one or several medical personnel (or sometimes commissions) are required.	Allow the woman to decide. If authorization is required by law, avoid multiple signatures or approval by a committee; assign responsibility to qualified persons who are readily available in the health system.	Approval by someone other than the woman is not medically indicated (except in rare circumstances when abortion would present a medical risk for the woman).
Time limits that are not medically indicated or in the law are imposed on length of pregnancy for which abortion is performed.	Revise or remove limits on the length of pregnancy that are not medically or legally required.	In some countries, for instance, a limit of 8 weeks is put on the performance of manual vacuum aspiration, whereas it can be used safely up to 12 weeks by trained providers.
Waiting period is required between request for and provision of abortion or clients are placed on a waiting list.	Eliminate waiting periods that are not medically required, and expand services to serve all eligible women promptly.	Waiting periods unnecessarily delay care and decrease safety.

Table 4.2 **Administrative and regulatory barriers to obtaining safe, legal abortion, and measures to eliminate these barriers** *continued*

Barriers	Possible actions	Rationale
Spousal authorization, or parental notification or authorization, is required.	If not required by law, ensure providers do not impose spousal or parental authorization. If required by law, in the case of minor, unmarried women, allow authorization by persons other than a parent, if the minor feels she cannot approach a parent (e.g. when the parent is abusive).	Such requirements deter women from seeking timely care and may lead them to risk self-induced abortion or clandestine services.
Certain groups of women are excluded from services by health care providers.	Allow all women eligible by law access to abortion services free of discrimination by marital status, age, or any other characteristic not required by law. Train providers not to discriminate, and sanction those who do.	International consensus documents recognise the right of individuals to have access to methods of their choice for regulating fertility which are not against the law.
Rape and incest victims are required to press charges against the aggressor, obtain police reports, court authorization, or complete other medically-unnecessary steps to qualify for abortion.	Minimize requirements, develop and use clear protocols to facilitate prompt referral and access to appropriate care. Train police, court officials and health care providers to understand the need for prompt and compassionate action and to coordinate their services.	Juridical requirements delay necessary care and increase the likelihood of unsafe abortion.
Unnecessary restrictions on kinds of facilities that provide abortion limit access for women eligible under national law.	To comply with the human right of non-discrimination, extend services that meet safety requirements so that all women eligible under national law have access, irrespective of residence, income or other factors.	Unnecessarily restricting service locations prevents women from accessing services early, raises costs, and may encourage women to seek care from local but unqualified providers.

Barriers	Possible actions	Rationale
Standards that over-medicalize abortion are required (e.g. mandatory use of ultrasound, inpatient facilities, general anaesthesia, operating theatre, etc.).	Remove requirements not medically indicated. Modify service guidelines and make sure training institutions follow them.	Over-medicalization raises costs, reduces availability of services, does not improve, and may even reduce, safety and quality of care.
Only physicians are trained to provide abortion.	Train midlevel providers to the extent allowed by law.	Especially in situations where doctor-patient ratios are low, this requirement prevents women from accessing services early, raises costs, and leads women to seek care from unqualified providers. Trained, midlevel providers (e.g. midwives) can perform manual vacuum aspiration safely, and provide medical methods of abortion.
Health professionals exempt themselves from abortion care on the basis of conscientious objection, but do not refer the woman to another provider.	Require any health professional who claims conscientious objection to follow professional ethical standards.	Professional ethical standards usually require health professionals to refer the woman to another willing and trained provider in the same, or an easily accessible, health facility. Where referral is not possible and the woman's life is at stake, require the health professional to provide abortion in accordance with national law.

Table 4.2 **Administrative and regulatory barriers to obtaining safe, legal abortion, and measures to eliminate these barriers** *continued*

Barriers	Possible actions	Rationale
Methods of abortion are limited unnecessarily.	Introduce all methods suited to the capabilities of the health system.	In some countries, for example, D&C is the only method used even though vacuum aspiration would be safer, less costly, and also suitable at all levels of the health system. Introduction of medical methods in addition to surgical methods would expand access.
Official and informal fees or other charges reduce access to services, especially by poor women and adolescents who do not have access to funds.	Develop and implement equitable cost-recovery schemes that ensure that those without money can access services. Set fees in line with costs and monitor and stop informal charges.	Lowering fees expands access. The cost of subsidies will likely be offset by savings achieved from reducing unsafe abortion and the cost of managing their complications.
Confidentiality is not assured.	Establish guidelines for confidentiality, train staff, monitor and ensure compliance. Modify record-keeping system so that women's identity is concealed. Ensure private space for counselling so that conversations cannot be overheard.	Confidentiality is a key principle of medical ethics; failure to guarantee confidentiality may lead women to seek an unqualified provider.

References

Alan Guttmacher Institute. (1999) *Sharing responsibility: women, society and abortion worldwide*. New York and Washington DC, Alan Guttmacher Institute.

Alvarez-Lajonchere C. (1989) Commentary on abortion law and practice in Cuba. *International Journal of Gynecology and Obstetrics* Supplement 3:93/95.

Berer M. (2000) Making abortions safe: a matter of good public health policy and practice. *Bulletin of the World Health Organization* 78:580-592.

Billings DL, Moreno C, Ramos C, González de León D, Ramirez R, Martinez LV and Díaz MR. (2002) Constructing access to legal abortion services in Mexico City. *Reproductive Health Matters* 10(19):87-95.

Gupte M, Bandewar S and Pisal H. (1997) Abortion needs of women in India: a case study of rural Maharashtra. *Reproductive Health Matters* 5(9):77-86.

Iyengar K and Iyengar SD. (2002) Elective abortion as a primary health service in rural India: experience with manual vacuum aspiration. *Reproductive Health Matters* 10(19):55-64.

Koster-Oyekan W. (1998) Why resort to illegal abortion in Zambia? Findings of a community-based study in Western Province. *Social Science and Medicine* 46:1303-1312.

Mundigo AI and Indriso C (eds). (1999) *Abortion in the developing world*. New Delhi, Vistaar Publications for the World Health Organization.

Oye-Adeniran BA, Umoh AV and Nnatu SNN. (2002) Complications of unsafe abortion: a case study and the need for abortion law reform in Nigeria. *Reproductive Health Matters* 10(19):19-22.

Rahman A, Katzive L and Henshaw SK. (1998) A global review of laws on induced abortion, 1985-1997. *International Family Planning Perspectives* 24:56-64.

United Nations. (1995) *Report of the International Conference on Population and Development, Cairo, 5-13 September 1994*. New York, United Nations. (Sales No. 95.XIII.18)

United Nations. (1996) *Report of the Fourth World Conference on Women, Beijing, 4-15 September 1995*. New York, United Nations. (Sales No. 96.IV.13)

United Nations. (1999) *Key actions for the further implementation of the Programme of Action of the International Conference on Population and Development*. New York, United Nations. (A/S-21/5/Add.1)

United Nations. (2001a) *Abortion policies: a global review. Volume I Afghanistan to France*. New York, United Nations. (ST/ESA/SER.A/187)

United Nations. (2001b) *Abortion policies: a global review. Volume II Gabon to Norway*. New York, United Nations. (ST/ESA/SER.A/191)

United Nations. (2002) *Abortion policies: a global review. Volume III Oman to Zimbabwe*. New York, United Nations. (ST/ESA/SER.A/196)

United Nations Population Division. (1999) *World abortion policies 1999*. New York, United Nations Population Division. (ST/ESA/SER.A/178)

Veira Villela W and de Oliveira Araujo MJ. (2000) Making legal abortion available in Brazil: partnerships in practice. *Reproductive Health Matters* 8(16):77-82.

World Health Organization. (1998) *Unsafe abortion: global and regional estimates of incidence of and mortality due to unsafe abortion with a listing of available country data*. Geneva, World Health Organization. (WHO/RHT/MSM/97.16)

World Health Organization. (2001) *Basic documents*. Forty-third edition. Geneva, World Health Organization.

Annex 1 Further reading and resources

American College of Obstetricians and Gynecologists. Domestic violence. ACOG educational bulletin. (2000) *International Journal of Gynecology and Obstetrics* 71:79-87.

Annett H and Rifkin S. (1995) *Guidelines for rapid participatory appraisals to assess community health needs.* Geneva, World Health Organization.

AVSC International. (1995) Postabortion women. In AVSC International. *Family planning counseling - a curriculum prototype.* New York, AVSC International.

AVSC International. (1999) *Infection prevention curriculum: a training course for health care providers and other staff of hospitals and clinics.* New York, AVSC International.

AVSC International. (2000) *Infection prevention: multimedia package (Training CD-ROM and reference booklet).* New York, AVSC International.

Baird DT, Grimes DA and Van Look PFA (eds). (1995) *Modern methods of inducing abortion.* Oxford, Blackwell Science.

Baird T, Castleman LD, Gringle RE and Blumenthal PD. (2000) *Clinician's guide for second-trimester abortion.* Carrboro, NC, Ipas.

Baird TL and Flinn SK. (2001) *Manual vacuum aspiration: expanding women's access to safe abortion services.* Chapel Hill, NC, Ipas.

Baker A. (1995) *Abortion and options counseling: a comprehensive reference.* Granite City, IL, The Hope Clinic for Women.

Bertrand J and Tsui A. (1995) *Indicators for reproductive health program evaluation.* Chapel Hill, NC, The Evaluation Project.

Brazier E, Rizzuto R and Wolf M. (1998) *Prevention and management of unsafe abortion: a guide for action.* New York, Family Care International.

Center for Reproductive Law and Policy. (2000) *Making abortion safe, legal, and accessible: a tool kit for action.* New York, Center for Reproductive Law and Policy.

Comprehensive abortion care with Ipas MVA Plus ™ - Reference manual and trainer's manual. Chapel Hill, NC, Ipas (forthcoming).

Consortium for Emergency Contraception. (2000) *Emergency contraceptive pills: medical and service delivery guidelines.* Seattle, Consortium for Emergency Contraception.

Consortium for Emergency Contraception. (2000) *Expanding global access to emergency contraception. A collaborative approach to meeting women's needs.* Seattle, Consortium for Emergency Contraception.

Cook R and Dickens B. (2001) *Advancing safe motherhood through human rights.* Geneva, World Health Organization. (WHO/RHR/01.5)

Cook RJ, Dickens BM and Bliss LE. (1999) International developments in abortion law from 1988 to 1998. *Amercian Journal of Public Health* 89:579-586.

Counseling the postabortion patient: training for service providers. Trainer's guide (draft). (1999) New York, AVSC International.

DataPAC Core Questionnaire Series. Final Report. (1998) Carrboro, NC, Ipas. (2001)

DeBruyn M. (2001) *Violence, pregnancy and abortion: issues of women's rights and public health. A review of worldwide data and recommendations for action.* Chapel Hill, NC, Ipas.

Dickson-Tetteh K, Gabriel M, Rees H, Gringle R and Winkler J. (1998) *Abortion care manual: a guide for the training of registered midwives in termination of pregnancy, management of incomplete abortion and related reproductive health matters.* Johannesburg, Reproductive Health Research Unit and Ipas.

Foreit R and Frejka T (eds). (1998) *Family planning operations research.* New York, Population Council.

Gerhardt AJ, Hausknecht R, Baird TL and Shochet T. (2000) *Manual vacuum aspiration. Slide presentation on one compact disc.* New York, Physicians for Reproductive Choice and Health.

Germain A and Kim T (1998) *Expanding access to safe abortion: strategies for action.* New York, International Women's Health Coalition.

Hord CE. (2001) *Making safe abortion accessible: a practical guide for advocates.* Chapel Hill, NC, Ipas.

Hord CE, Baird TL and Billings DL. (1999) *Advancing the role of midlevel providers in abortion and postabortion care: a global review and key future actions.* Issues in Abortion Care No. 6. Carrboro, NC, Ipas.

Huber D. (1997) *Postpartum and postabortion contraception: a comprehensive training course.* Watertown, MA, Pathfinder International.

Paul M, Lichtenberg ES, Borgatta L, Grimes D and Stubblefield PG (eds). (1999) *A clinician's guide to medical and surgical abortion.* Philadelphia, Churchill Livingstone.

Pereira IG and Novaes da Mota C. (2000) *Manual para o estabelecimento de um servico de atendimento para aborto previsto por lei [Manual for establishing services for providing abortion foreseen by law].* Carrboro, NC, Ipas.

Physicians for Reproductive Choice and Health. (1999) *Medical abortion slide and lecture presentation.* New York, Physicians for Reproductive Choice and Health.

Policar MJ and Pollack AE. (1995) *Clinical training curriculum in abortion practice.* Washington, DC, National Abortion Federation.

Reproductive Health for Refugees Consortium. (1997) *Refugee reproductive health needs assessment field tools.* New York, RHR Consortium.

Reproductive Health for Refugees Consortium. (1998) *Five-day training program for health personnel on reproductive health programming in refugee settings.* New York, RHR Consortium.

Rinehart W, Rudy S and Drenna M. (1998) *GATHER guide to counseling.* Population Reports, Series J, No. 48. Baltimore, Johns Hopkins University School of Public Health, Population Information Program.

Santana F, Sloan NL, Schiavon R, Billings D, King T, Pobia, B and Langer A. (2000) *Guidelines and instructions for monitoring and evaluation of postabortion care services (electronic version 1.0).* New York, The Population Council.

Solter C, Farrell B and Gutierrez M. (1997) *Manual vacuum aspiration: a comprehensive training course.* Watertown, MA, Pathfinder International.

Talluri-Rao S and Baird TL. (1999) *Counseling and information guide for medical abortion – with training guide.* Chapel Hill, NC, Ipas.

United Nations Office of the High Commissioner for Human Rights. For further information related to International Human Rights Covenants, Conventions and other documents see: *www.unhchr.ch.*

Varkey SJ, Fonn S and Ketlhapile M. (2001) *Health workers for choice: working to improve quality of abortion services.* Johannesburg, Women's Health Project, University of the Witwatersrand.

WHO Certification scheme on the quality of pharmaceutical products moving in international commerce. For online information see *www.who.int/medicines/library/dap.*

Winkler J and Gringle R. (1999) *Postabortion family planning: a two day curriculum for improving counseling and services.* Chapel Hill, NC, Ipas.

Wolf M and Benson J. (1994) Meeting women's needs for postabortion family planning: report of a Bellagio technical working group. *International Journal of Gynecology and Obstetrics* 45 (Supplement).

World Health Organization. (1995) *Complications of abortion: technical and managerial guidelines for prevention and treatment.* Geneva, World Health Organization.

World Health Organization. (1996) *Studying unsafe abortion: a practical guide.* Geneva, World Health Organization. (WHO/RHT/MSM/96.25)

Annex 1 Further reading and resources *continued*

World Health Organization. (1997) *Post-abortion family planning: a practical guide for programme managers.* Geneva, World Health Organization. (WHO/RHT/97.20)

World Health Organization. (1999) *Interpreting reproductive health.* Geneva, World Health Organization. (WHO/CHS/RHR/99.7)

World Health Organization. (2000) *Strengthening the provision of adolescent friendly health services to meet the health and development needs of adolescents in Africa. A consensus statement.* Geneva, World Health Organization. (WHO/FCH/CAH/01.16 and AFR/ADH/01.3)

Yordy L, Leonard AH and Winkler J. (1993) *Manual vacuum aspiration guide for clinicians.* Carrboro, NC, Ipas.

Annex 2 International consensus documents in relation to safe abortion

In recent decades, international understanding of the basic civil, social and economic rights with which all people are born has deepened and been progressively articulated in international covenants, treaties and other instruments. Such agreements create a solid basis for real improvements in people's lives, as ratifying nations commit themselves to uphold the rights enumerated therein, including by adjusting laws and policies.

The series of International Conferences which took place during the decade of the 1990s developed documents which elaborate on the aspects of reproductive health. These international consensus documents which have been adopted by the majority of countries have the backing of the Human Rights Treaty Bodies' framework, and have been most explicit in articulating rights in relation to reproductive health. Below are statements from recent international consensus documents that highlight issues relevant to safe abortion.

1974   World Population Conference,
        Bucharest Plan of Action
"All couples and individuals have the basic right to decide freely and responsibly the number and spacing of their children and to have the information, education and means to do so."
Paragraph 14(f)

1984 Recommendations for the Further Implementation of the World Population Plan of Action, Mexico City

"The World Population Plan of Action recognizes, as one of its principles, the basic human right of all couples and individuals to decide freely and responsibly the number and spacing of their children. For this right to be realized, couples and individuals must have access to the necessary education, information and means to regulate their fertility, regardless of the overall demographic goals of the Government."

Paragraph 24

1994 Programme of Action Adopted at the International Conference on Population and Development, Cairo

"Advancing gender equality and equity and the empowerment of women ... and ensuring women's ability to control their own fertility are cornerstones of population and development-related programmes."

Principle 4

"Reproductive health is a state of complete physical, mental and social well-being and not merely the absence of disease or infirmity, in all matters relating to the reproductive system and to its functions and processes. Reproductive health therefore implies that people are able to have a satisfying and safe sex life and that they have the capability to reproduce and the freedom to decide if, when and how often to do so.

Implicit in this last condition are the rights of men and women to be informed and to have access to safe, effective, affordable, and acceptable methods of family planning of their choice, as well as other methods of their choice for regulation of fertility which are not against the law..."

Paragraph 7.2

"[R]eproductive rights embrace certain human rights that are already recognized in national laws, international human rights documents and other consensus documents. These rights rest on the recognition of the basic right of all couples and individuals to decide freely and responsibly the number, spacing and timing of their children and to have the information and means to do so, and the right to attain the highest standard of sexual and reproductive health. It also includes their right to make decisions concerning reproduction free of discrimination, coercion and violence ... The promotion of the responsible exercise of these [reproductive] rights should be the fundamental basis for government- and community-supported policies and programmes in the area of reproductive health, including family planning."

Paragraph 7.3

"[G]overnments should make it easier for couples and individuals to take responsibility for their own reproductive health by removing unnecessary legal, medical, clinical and regulatory barriers to information and to access to family-planning services and methods."

Paragraph 7.20

"In no case should abortion be promoted as a method of family planning. All Governments and relevant intergovernmental and non-governmental organizations are urged to strengthen their commitment to women's health, to deal with the health impact of unsafe abortion* as a major public health concern and to reduce the recourse to abortion through expanded and improved family planning services. Prevention of unwanted pregnancies must always be given the highest priority and all attempts should be made to eliminate the need for abortion. Women who have unwanted pregnancies should have ready access to reliable information and compassionate counseling. Any measures or changes related to abortion within the health system can only be determined at the national or local level according to the national legislative process. In circumstances in which abortion is not against the law, such abortion should be safe. In all cases women should have access to quality services for the management of complications arising from abortion. Postabortion counseling, education and family planning services should be offered promptly which will also help to avoid repeat abortions.

*Unsafe abortion is defined as a procedure for terminating an unwanted pregnancy either by persons lacking the necessary skills or in an environment lacking the minimal medical standards or both. (WHO)"
Paragraph 8.25

1995   Fourth World Conference on Women, Beijing
"The human rights of women include their right to have control over and decide freely and responsibly on matters related to their sexuality, including sexual and reproductive health, free of coercion, discrimination and violence. Equal relationships between women and men in matters of sexual relations and reproduction, including full respect for the integrity of the person, require mutual respect, consent and shared responsibility for sexual behaviour and its consequences."
Paragraph 96

"Governments, in collaboration with non-governmental organizations and employers' and workers' organizations and with the support of international institutions [should]:

j.   Recognize and deal with the health impact of unsafe abortion as a major public health concern, as agreed in paragraph 8.25 of the Programme of Action of the International Conference on Population and Development;

k.   In the light of paragraph 8.25 of the Programme of Action of the International Conference on Population and Development... consider reviewing laws containing punitive measures against women who have undergone illegal abortions."
Paragraph 106

1999 Key Actions for the Further Implementation of the Programme of Action of the International Conference on Population and Development

"(i) In no case should abortion be promoted as a method of family planning. All Governments and relevant intergovernmental and non-governmental organizations are urged to strengthen their commitment to women's health, to deal with the health impact of unsafe abortion as a major public-health concern and to reduce the recourse to abortion through expanded and improved family planning services. Prevention of unwanted pregnancies must always be given the highest priority and every attempt should be made to eliminate the need for abortion. Women who have unwanted pregnancies should have ready access to reliable information and compassionate counselling. Any measures or changes related to abortion within the health system can only be determined at the national or local level according to the national legislative process. In circumstances where abortion is not against the law, such abortion should be safe. In all cases, women should have access to quality services for the management of complications arising from abortion. Post-abortion counselling, education and family planning services should be offered promptly, which will also help to avoid repeat abortions.

(ii) Governments should take appropriate steps to help women avoid abortion, which in no case should be promoted as a method of family planning, and in all cases provide for the humane treatment and counselling of women who have had recourse to abortion.

(iii) In recognizing and implementing the above, and in circumstances where abortion is not against the law, health systems should train and equip health-service providers and should take other measures to ensure that such abortion is safe and accessible. Additional measures should be taken to safeguard women's health."
Paragraph 63

2000 Further Actions and Initiatives to implement the Beijing Declaration and the Platform for Action

"Design and implement programmes with the full involvement of adolescents as appropriate, to provide them with education, information and appropriate, specific, user-friendly and accessible services without discrimination to address effectively their reproductive and sexual health needs taking into account their right to privacy, confidentiality, respect and informed consent and the responsibilities, rights and duties of parents and legal guardians to provide in a manner consistent with the evolving capacities of the child appropriate direction and guidance in the exercise by the child of the rights recognized in the Convention on the Rights of the Child and in conformity with CEDAW and ensuring that in all actions concerning children, the best interests of the child are a primary consideration."
Paragraph 115fbis

Annex 3 Instruments and supplies for manual vacuum aspiration (MVA)

Basic Supplies

- intravenous infusion set and fluids (sodium lactate, glucose, saline)

- aspirators (syringes) (5, 10 and 20 ml)

- needles (22 gauge spinal for paracervical block; 21 gauge for drug administration)

- sterile gloves (small, medium, large)

- cotton swabs or gauze sponges

- water-based antiseptic solution (not alcohol-based)

- detergent or soap

- clean water

- chlorine or glutaraldehyde for disinfection/decontamination

- high-level disinfection or sterilization agent

Instruments and Equipment

- vaginal speculum

- tenaculum

- sponge (ring) forceps or uterine packing forceps

- Pratt or Denniston dilators: sizes 13 to 27 French

- container for antiseptic solution

- strainer (metal, glass, or gauze)

- clear glass dish for tissue inspection

Medications

- analgesia medication (e.g. acetaminophen, ibuprofen, or pethidine)

- anti-anxiety medication (e.g. diazepam)

- anaesthetic – chloroprocaine (1-2%) or lidocaine (0.5-2%) without epinephrine

- oxytocin 10 units or ergometrine 0.2mg

MVA Instruments

- vacuum aspirator

- flexible cannulae of different sizes

- adapters, if needed

- silicone for lubricating syringes, if needed

Annex 4 Contraception following abortion

Method	Timing after Abortion	Remarks
Oral Contraceptives (combined and progestogen-only pills)	▪ can start combined or progestogen-only pill use immediately, including on the day of procedure	▪ if adequate counselling and informed decision-making cannot be guaranteed, delay starting pills and provide condoms in the meantime ▪ no protection against STI/HIV infection ▪ can be started immediately, even if infection is present
Injectables (DMPA, NET-EN, Cyclofem and Mesigyna)	▪ may be given immediately	▪ if adequate counselling and informed decision-making cannot be guaranteed, delay first injection and provide condoms in the meantime ▪ no protection against STI/HIV ▪ can be started immediately, even if infection is present
Implants	▪ may be given immediately	▪ if adequate counselling and informed decision-making cannot be guaranteed, delay insertion and provide condoms in the meantime ▪ access to a provider skilled in insertion and removal is necessary ▪ no protection against STI/HIV ▪ can be started immediately, even if infection is present

Method	Timing after Abortion	Remarks
IUD	• IUDs can be inserted if risk or presence of infection can be ruled out • delay insertion until serious injury is healed, haemorrhage is controlled and acute anaemia improves	• if adequate counselling and informed decision-making cannot be guaranteed, delay insertion and provide condoms in the meantime • access to a provider skilled in insertion and removal is necessary • no protection against STI/HIV • there is some concern about a greater risk of expulsion after second trimester abortion • uterine perforation can occur during insertion • if infection is present, IUD should not be inserted for at least 3 months after abortion procedure
Condoms (male or female)	• start as soon as intercourse is resumed	• good interim method if another method is chosen but cannot be started immediately; good continuing method if used consistently and correctly • male condom is the only method proven to provide protection against both pregnancy and STI/HIV • female condom helps to protect against HIV/STI, but may be less effective than the male condom

Method	Timing after Abortion	Remarks
Spermicides (foam, cream, film, jelly, suppositories, tablets)	▪ start as soon as intercourse is resumed	▪ possible interim method if initiation of another method must be postponed ▪ substantially less effective than other methods ▪ no protection against STI/HIV
Barrier Methods (diaphragm used with spermicide; cervical cap)	▪ diaphragm can be fitted immediately after first trimester abortion ▪ after second trimester abortion, diaphragm fitting should be delayed until uterus returns to pre-pregnancy size (in 6 weeks) ▪ fitting of cervical cap should be delayed until uterus returns to pre-pregnancy size (4-6 weeks)	▪ diaphragm fitted prior to a second trimester abortion may be too small immediately after procedure due to change in the vaginal tissue and/or cervix ▪ diaphragm may provide some protection against STIs; protection against HIV should not be assumed
Fertility Awareness-Based Methods	▪ not recommended for immediate post-abortion use ▪ women can use as soon as they have completed 3 post-abortion menses	▪ effectiveness is highly dependent on proper use ▪ no protection against STI/HIV

Annex 4 Contraception following abortion *continued*

Method	Timing after Abortion	Remarks
Tubal Occlusion	• tubal occlusion (mini laparotomy or laparoscopy) can be performed immediately after an uncomplicated abortion • in cases of post-abortal sepsis or fever, severe post-abortal haemorrhage, severe trauma to the genital tract, or acute haematometra, the procedure must be delayed until satisfactory treatment has been completed and/or injury has healed	• adequate counselling and informed decision-making and consent must take place before voluntary sterilization procedures (tubal occlusion or vasectomy) • no protection against STI/HIV
Emergency Contraceptive Pills (levonorgestrel-only and combined estrogen-progestogen regimens)	• can be used as soon as unprotected intercourse takes place	• not suitable as regular method of contraception • important back-up method following unprotected intercourse • no protection against STI/HIV

Source: The information in this table is based on: World Health Organization. (2000) *Improving access to quality care in family planning - Medical eligibility criteria for contraceptive use.* Second edition. Geneva, World Health Organization. (WHO/RHR/00.2)